SO-ANE-334

Working After Brain Injury:

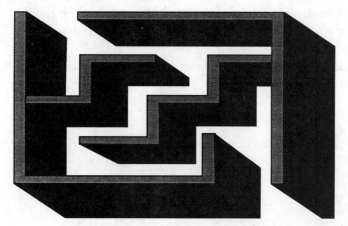

What Can I Do?

Dana S. DeBoskey, Ph.D., Editor
With
John T. Burton, M.S.
Connie J. Calub, M.Ed.
Karen Morin, M.S.W.

© Copyright 1996

No part of this book may be reproduced, stored in a retrieval system, or transmitted, by any means, electronic or mechanical, including photocopying, without written permission from the publisher.

Printed in the United States of America on acid free paper. ∞

Library of Congress Cataloging-in-Publication Data
Working after brain injury what can I do? / Dana S. DeBoskey,
    editor.
        p.   cm.
        ISBN 1-882855-35-3
        1. Brain damage--Patients--Employment. 2. Brain damage--
Patients--Rehabilitation. 3. Occupational therapy. I. DeBoskey,
Dana S.
RC387.5.W67   1996
617.4'81044--dc20

                                                                      96-2421
                                                                       CIP

WORKING AFTER BRAIN INJURY: WHAT CAN I DO?

This manual was developed and produced by DeBoskey and Associates, Tampa, Florida. Other volumes by DeBoskey and Associates published by HDI include:

Coming Home: A Discharge Manual for Families of Persons with a Brain Injury

An Educational Challenge: Meeting the Needs of Students with Brain Injury

Pain: Making Life Liveable

Dana S. DeBoskey, Editor
with
John T. Burton, M.S.
Connie J. Calub, M.Ed.
Karen Morin, M.S.W.
and
HDI staff members
Linda L. Thoi, M.P.H.
Beth L. Droll
Bonnie J. Haynes

For a complete catalog of HDI's brain injury resources contact:

HDI Publishers
P.O. Box 131401
Houston, TX 77219-1401
Toll Free (800) 321-7037
(713) 682-8700
Fax (713) 956-2288

© 1996 HDI Publishers

TABLE OF CONTENTS

PREFACE

Often one of the first coherent requests that is formulated by the person who is brain injured is "When can I go back to work?" For many this thought is foremost in their mind. Returning to work is considered synonymous with "getting better" or, better still, "being normal again." It is definitely a very important benchmark in the rehabilitation process. There are, however, many steps that must precede an effective and efficient effort to return to work. These would involve acute inpatient rehabilitation, as well as outpatient therapy that includes day treatment cognitive rehabilitation and psychosocial skills groups. From here an individual would receive a work evaluation and/or further vocational testing to determine the most appropriate job placement. For other groups of individuals who are disabled the only remaining problem would be finding the job. However, for the population of the brain injured there is an even greater hurdle - keeping the job. This difficulty occurs at a much higher rate than with other rehabilitation populations due to the large variety of cognitive and behavioral problems that result from damage to the brain. These deficit areas are the focus of the manual. The primary audience is the person who is brain injured; however, the information can also be used as a guide by vocational counselors, job coaches, rehabilitation providers, and psychotherapists.

Dana S. DeBoskey, Ph.D.
Clinical Director
DeBoskey and Associates
March, 1996

I. INTRODUCTION

Many of us associate "what we do" with "who we are." When you meet a new acquaintance in a social gathering a common question arises..."And what do *you* do?" They are not asking "What do you do when someone needs help?" or "What do you do on the weekends?" of course. They mean "What do you do for a living?"

For some individuals this question is merely a conversation opener, and the person asking may not be greatly interested in your work. For others, this is a method of evaluating you. Do you have a desk job, construction job, sales job, or managerial position? If you have been out of work for a considerable length of time you have probably faced this question and, in fact, answered it in a variety of ways. We can empathize with the various reactions you have gotten when you admitted to the current situation.

This manual is written for all the individuals with a brain injury who hope to go back to work, who are ready to go back to work, who may have tried to work and failed, and who are ready to try again. There are a multitude of barriers to returning to the work force, including physical problems, cognitive (thinking) problems, emotional (feeling) problems, and behavior (acting) problems.

We will leave the solely physical issues to physicians, physical therapists, and occupational therapists; however, the cognitive and emotional difficulties will be discussed in detail.

We have set forth a very comprehensive list of all the problems that could possibly arise in these areas. Please do not conclude that we are saying you must be having all of these difficulties.

As you well know, if you have had the opportunity to socialize with other people who are brain injured, deficit areas vary significantly in both severity and frequency. In an effort to provide complete information, we have included all of the possible things that could go wrong.

It is also hoped that you will not perceive that we are presenting individuals with a brain injury solely as a group of people with multiple negative characteristics. We are very aware of all the positive gains that you must have made from the time of injury to now. All of the authors have worked with numerous individuals who are brain injured in helping them in their re-entry into community life. We have followed some people for five years or more and are, thus, quite aware of the multitude of issues that arise. In order to comprehensively address these issues, we have listed everything that might be negative so that we can provide positive ways to approach the problems. For each area we have briefly described the issue, presented real life examples, and offered a menu-type listing of approaches to try. Please do not be discouraged if you try some of the suggestions and they do not bring the desired results. Move on to another idea or ask a professional to help you evaluate your efforts.

This book is written for you - the person with a brain injury. Others may find it helpful in understanding your struggle to return to work; however, it is written to provide you with ideas for change. The authors are fully aware that not all individuals who are brain injured are male. Nevertheless, for the sake of simplicity we have used the pronoun he to represent all those returning to work. We hope this will not be offensive to any of our readers.

II. THINKING ISSUES ON THE JOB

As you well know, having a brain injury yourself, there are a multitude of problems that can follow the injury. Many of these difficulties may have been quite evident to you, such as motor problems and other physical inadequencies. On the other hand, some of the more subtle deficits are harder for you to recognize. These are often cognitive or thinking difficulties.

If your injury was a brain injury that resulted in no skull fracture, hematoma (bruise) or surgical opening of the skull, it may be even more difficult for you to imagine that your brain has been affected to the point that you do not think exactly as you did prior to the incident. However, even a mild blow to the head resulting in less than 20 minutes of unconsciousness can lead to headaches, memory problems, poor concentration, and general confusion.

How does this happen? When your accident occurred your brain was shaken up inside the skull. There is no place for the brain to go so it jiggles back and forth against the inside walls of the skull. Inside your skull there are some rough boney surfaces that can bruise the areas of the brain next to them. These parts of the brain are the sites just above the ears (temporal lobes) and the bottom part of the forehead area (frontal lobes). These areas are very important in many cognitive or thinking abilities such as attention, concentration, memory, problem solving, and impulsivity.

You may think that you do not have these difficulties if pictures of your brain (CAT SCAN or MRI) or recordings of your brain waves (EEG) have indicated normal results. Abnormal readings of these measures are evidence that problems exist; however, normal readings do not rule out the existence of more subtle abnormalities that can lead to thinking problems. Axons in the brain can be sheared or broken causing subtle difficulties in processing information that you either see or hear. These axons can regenerate, but they may or may not make the appropriate connections. This can lead to faulty thinking, inaccurate interpretation of information, and/or expressive problems.

At this point you may be thinking, "What's the use? If I have brain damage I can't work." That is definitely not the case. There are many individuals with varying degrees of brain injury who are quite capable of employment. The trick is to compensate or make up for your weaknesses, and be willing to look at work options that capitalize on your assets and minimize your problems.

Following are listed a multitude of thinking problems that may interfere with your return to the workforce. You may feel that only a few of them apply to you. Nevertheless, we recommend that you read through all sections just to familiarize yourself with the potential difficulties. It may be that once you are in a work setting a problem may arise that you were not aware of before returning to work. The skills required on a particular job may be very different from those required at home or in previous job settings.

Depending upon your work environment and/or your immediate supervisor, you may want to share some of the information that is pertinent to you with your employer. This would have to be an individualized decision based upon your particular circumstances. If you are unsure as to the feasibility or helpfulness of doing this, consult a family member or therapist with whom you maintain contact.

A. REMEMBERING WHAT TO DO AND WHEN TO DO IT

Memory problems are probably the most well known or advertised thinking deficits in the area of brain injury. Even if you have had a mild head injury you may have experienced a reduction in your ability to remember. There are different types of memory as well as different levels of effect.

First, you may have problems with visual memory (taking in information through your eyes), or difficulty with auditory memory (taking in information through your ears). Secondly, you may not be able to get information into your brain easily (encoding) or, if it goes in, you may not be able to find it later (retrieval). Third, you may be one of those people who can remember things better if you do not have to deal with another task that would interfere and lead to forgetting the first task. Fourth, you may be able to learn something only if you go over it many, many times so that it can become automatic.

If you are reading this book at the request of a therapist or rehabilitation specialist who is attempting to help you get back into the job market, we will assume that you have obtained, or are in the process of receiving, rehabilitation of your cognitive or thinking deficits. This book is not set up to provide suggestions for correcting your memory problems. Instead it is designed to provide you with methods of dealing with those problems.

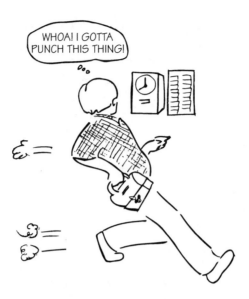

Examples

1. When you go to work in the morning you seem to be able to remember to punch the time clock on the way in. However, when leaving for the day you are forgetting to clock out at least 2-3 times a week.

2. Your boss is constantly saying he is sure he told you something about which you have no recollection.

3. In your job as a service manager in a car dealership you find that you are frequently overbooked with customers who bring their cars in for service and you are sure you never spoke to them on the phone.

4. Even though you have met the salesmen in your store many times, you confuse their names and faces.

5. In your job as a building contractor you are constantly setting the blue prints down some-

where and then having difficulty locating them.

Compensation Techniques

1. Carry a notebook with you at all times so that you can record all information that should be stored in your brain. There are many types of organizers that have calendars, as well as additional sections for recording and storing lists of things to do, contacts with individuals, addresses, and phone numbers, and ideas for new or old projects.

2. Ask a professional to tell you exactly what processes of memory are the most difficult for you. For example, if your visual memory is intact, but you have difficulty with remembering things that you hear, you can adjust for this by a) asking your boss to always show you how to do something the first time rather than just telling you, b) writing down instructions, and c) taking notes at staff meetings.

3. Never be embarrassed to use any technique that has been suggested. There are many individuals who have not been injured who need to do this.

4. Never try to cover up for your problem by being unwilling to consult a colleague about something you have forgotten.

5. Although there is a slim possibility that fellow workers could use your memory problems to cover up their inadequencies, this situation would rarely be the case. Instead, you must allow yourself to believe people are telling you the truth about your forgetfulness.

6.   Sometimes you will not hear about the inadequencies of your memory difficulties until the boss is proposing that you be terminated. Don't let it go this far. Periodically ask either your boss or a fellow co-worker if they see your memory causing problems on the job.

7.   Set up a large bulletin board over your desk so that you can post constant reminders for yourself.

8.   Xerox important papers that have a high probability of getting misplaced.

9.   Have a designated place to put away important things in your work space.

B. CONCENTRATING AND PAYING ATTENTION

Sometimes the memory problems described in the previous section are in part due to difficulty concentrating. Because you are not giving your absolute attention to the task at hand, you may find that you are totally forgetting, performing carelessly, or missing parts of information.

As an individual who is brain injured it is important for you to recognize this deficit and agree to minimize the consequences. You must constantly remind yourself to be a good listener and observer. In addition, it is very important to have a work area that is free from visual and/or auditory distractions. Brain injury makes it difficult for you to filter out many of the extraneous activities that go on around you on the job.

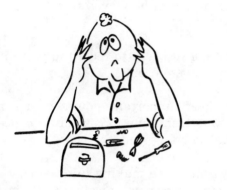

Examples

1. The constant clatter of machinery makes it difficult for you to effectively assemble your computer boards.

2. When people are standing behind your desk carrying on a conversation you have extreme problems focusing on your work task.

3. Before the injury you used to be able to study all morning without a break. Now you have to get up and walk around at least every twenty minutes.

4. You find that your mind frequently wanders out the window and your thoughts turn to projected activities for the weekend.

5. While sitting in a meeting you miss hearing what the boss is saying because you are frantically writing down what he said earlier.

Compensation Techniques

1. Minimize all outside distractors in your work area.

2. If your desk can be moved to a less congested area - do it.

3. Use a tape recorder to record important meetings or conversations.

4. Write down important points of a conversation - this technique forces you to concentrate on what is being said.

5. If co-workers are making unnecessary conversation in your space, nicely ask them to converse elsewhere.

6. Maintain eye contact with individuals who are talking to you on the job.

7. If something seems out of line check over your work to see if you have made a careless error - better still, always check your work.

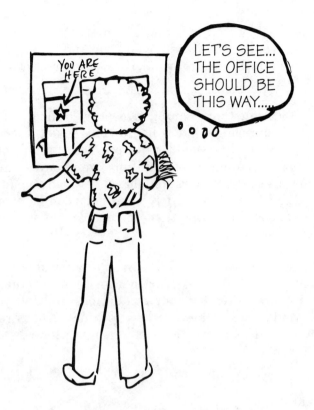

C. PERCEIVING CORRECTLY

After brain injury some individuals have difficulty with what is called visual perception, or the ability to perceive visual material accurately. Sometimes people will think this means they need glasses; however, it is not related to visual acuity or your ability to accurately see through your eyes. Instead, it has to do with how your brain interprets that visual material and then allows you to make decisions based on what you "think" you see.

Another form of perception is the ability to see where you are within an area and to be able to relate this to the total environment. Sometimes you may think you have difficulty finding a place that you have been to before because of your memory problem. Memory may be a factor, but this problem could also stem from difficulty with visual/spatial perception. You are not able to visualize in your mind where you are and, therefore, have a hard time remembering the directions in the future.

Still another form of perceptual difficulties is that of confusing what is heard. This is not a hearing problem that would require a hearing aid, but is, instead, a matter of "thinking" you heard something else. It is understandable that this can cause much confusion on the job. Directions can be interpreted so differently that the whole job is completed incorrectly.

If you are not sure if this is a noticeable area of deficit for you, ask your therapists or vocational counselors to review your evaluations and tell you the findings. If it has not been evaluated, it is recommended you have a brief screening for perceptual problems.

Examples

1.   You were a master auto mechanic prior to the accident, but now you have difficulty completing a repair job because at times you do not recognize various auto parts and are unsure exactly where they go.

2.   Reading blueprints is no longer second nature to you.

3.   You have difficulty remembering the truck routes you used to travel without consulting a map.

4.   You have to carry with you at all times a map of the large warehouse as you constantly take a wrong turn when delivering interoffice mail.

5. It used to take only 20 minutes to make out everybody's work schedule for the week. Now it takes closer to two hours.

6. Charts and graphs are very difficult to interpret.

7. You have difficulty determining the best way to revamp the filing system that your boss has asked you to update for months.

8. You spend hours xeroxing three entire books when all that your boss wanted was three pages from one book.

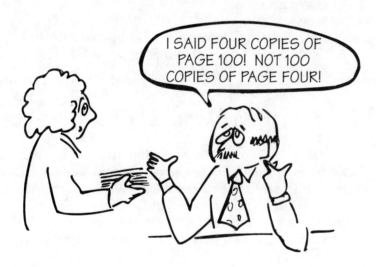

Compensation Techniques

1. Ask your boss or supervisor to always provide you with a verbal explanation of all visual materials in the job.

2. Try to devise cues to remember how to get to places that you find difficult to locate.

3. When you park your car in a mall or any type of parking garage, record in your wallet or purse the location of your vehicle.

4. Before you go on a' job related trip (or even one for enjoyment), make sure you determine exactly how to get there. Do not be afraid to stop and ask before you have gone too far out of your way.

5. When you are asked to visually organize a task, give yourself ample time to complete it so that you can allow for any confusion you may encounter.

6. Ask a trusted co-worker to help you with difficult perception tasks or to, at least, check over what you have completed.

D. INITIATING A TASK

Do you find yourself having trouble getting started on a task? Do you avoid certain job activities at all cost? Do you consider yourself lazy? After a brain injury many individuals have a difficult time initiating an activity and the end result is procrastination. You may be able to get away with this at home, but it will definitely cause problems on the job.

Instead of thinking of yourself as lazy, let's look at the reasons for this feeling of inertia. Due to a variety of cognitive problems experienced by survivors of brain injury, many of the skills needed to start a project are lacking. You may have difficulty breaking the task down into parts. You may be confused about where to start. You may have a fear of failing so, in this case, it might be better

not to start than to start and fail. All of these issues can result in a job task that never gets off the
ground.

Your first job is to understand what is going
on with this initiation deficit, and then to make an
organized effort to jump in with both feet and
counteract the tendency to avoid the job activity.

Examples

1. Your boss asks you to develop a marketing
    plan for the new product they are considering
    and you have no idea where to begin.

2. The files need to be reorganized, but you can
    not quite figure out the best system to use -
    so you put it off for another day.

3. You have been asked to develop a mailing list
    that is a combination of six or seven other
    lists with some possible overlap. You find it
    difficult to determine the best way to organize
    or categorize the names.

4. Your boss asks you to phone around town and
    find the best price for a used part. You have
    trouble making the comparisons based upon
    price and condition, so you stop after a few
    calls.

5. You are finding it very difficult to consis-
    tently get up early since you have returned to
    work.

6. At the end of a work day you find that you
    have only accomplished 25% of what you
    planned to do.

7. You find yourself not following up on job interviews that have been set by your vocational rehabilitation counselor.

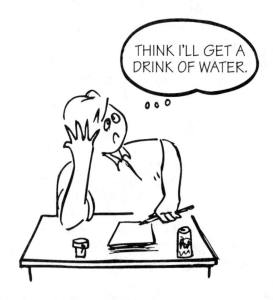

Compensation Techniques

1. Never let yourself put off until tomorrow what you can do today.

2. Set your goals for the day and try to accomplish at least 75% of them.

3. When you find yourself unable to plan a task, get help from an understanding supervisor or co-worker.

4. Do not let yourself commit to lots of projects at the same time. Additional stress will only make it difficult for you to accomplish each task.

5. Organize your work day in a calendar that includes a place to record your activities for the day.

6.   Once you have successfully completed a task on the job, do not just rest and wait to be told what to do next - ask what you need to do or, better still, start another project on your own.

E. COMPREHENDING WHAT IS SAID OR ASKED

Do co-workers tell you that the boss meant something different from what you thought? Do you find that your wife insists that she explained she would have to be away one week in June to a conference, and all you remember is her telling you she would like to go - not that she already signed up!

It is possible that your hearing and/or memory are adequate, but that you are misinterpreting the overall message. This occurs for various reasons, but is usually due to higher level processing skills that are not allowing for full comprehension of what you hear. Moreover, you may be listening only to what someone says and not noticing the gleam in their eye, the wink of their eye, or the presentation of some other type of nonverbal behavior that would negate the words they are speaking. I bet you are thinking "Well, people ought to say what they mean and, if they do not, it's not my fault." At first, you can tell your boss or co-workers to be straightforward with you, but ultimately you will want to relearn the subtle ways that people have of communicating.

Examples

1.   You are talking with your co-workers on break and someone asks you a question that seems totally unrelated to what you are all talking about.

2. It always seems like people are talking too fast.

3. Everyone at work laughs their head off every-time a co-worker opens his mouth. You some-times fake a laugh, but usually you do not see what is so funny. .

4. It is very difficult for you to learn something from a videotape.

5. You have read a memo and find that your co-worker has a completely different interpreta-tion of its content.

Compensation Techniques

1. Ask your supervisor to visually show you "how to" do a task instead of just telling you or having you read it in a manual.

2. Try to always double-check your interpreta-tion of an important conversation on the job.

3. Be a great listener - ask questions for clarifi-cation.

4. Ask for a review of the meeting and take some notes on important points or issues.

5. Never be embarrassed to ask someone to re-peat what they just said. You have to make sure you understand the issues initially or you will continue to misunderstand.

6. Accept the fact that you may not be 100% cor-rect all the time - you are a changed individ-ual - but this does not mean that you cannot develop good compensation strategies to util-ize on the job.

F. EXPRESSING MYSELF EASILY

You may frequently know what you want to say, but have trouble putting it on paper or in expressing it verbally. If you are lucky enough to have one of these methods spared, then you should definitely use it to either avoid or compensate for the weak area.

When you are considering going back to work you need to carefully analyze the skills that are needed for the prospective job. If you have difficulty with verbal expression, then it would be best to stay away from a job that requires constant verbal interaction with the public, particularly if this is a weak area that causes embarrassment for you. On the other hand, by forcing yourself to engage in this verbal discourse, you may be able to gain more confidence and cognitive skill. It is difficult to decide when you should give into your deficit areas and avoid jobs that require those skills, and when you should hit the deficit areas head on and make yourself overcome them or, at least, get more comfortable with them.

A therapist such as a speech/language pathologist, cognitive rehabilitation therapist, or neuropsychologist can help you decide between modifying your job capabilities or continuing to seek greater performance in verbal or written expression.

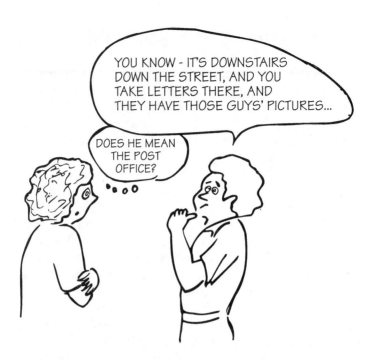

Examples

1. When you go to say something to your boss or supervisor, you have a hard time coming up with the most appropriate words to express yourself.

2. Finishing the necessary paperwork is very difficult for you - it seems to take so much longer.

3. It takes you 2-3 hours to prepare a menu, whereas prior to the injury you could whip one out in 20 minutes.

4. You find it very difficult to argue your point even when you and others are convinced you are correct in your thinking.

5. Your best friend at work says that you often ramble and never get to the point.

6. You always think of great things after the fact that you could have said when your supervisor challenged you on why you organized a job a certain way.

Compensation Techniques

1. If you have trouble putting your thoughts in written form, use a tape recorder and ask your boss to have your tape transcribed.

2. When you know you are going to meet with your boss or co-worker, think through what you want to say and how you want to express yourself. You can even role play with your spouse or other family member to make sure you get some practice. This should provide you with some self-confidence for expression.

3. If you are concerned that your written reports at work may have errors, ask a fellow co-worker to take a minute and look over your paperwork.

4. Never be embarrassed to reveal your shortcomings in this area. You will be respected for recognizing them and asking for assistance rather than pretending they do not exist.

5. If you do not think you have any expressive problems (verbal or written), you might want to double-check this perception with your supervisor. Be sure to tell them that you want honest feedback.

G. ACTING BEFORE THINKING

Have there been times when you have said something that later seemed quite wrong or inappropriate? You may have asked yourself "Why did I do that?" It may seem as if things just slip out without you thinking about it. If they do, your filtering system (the system that tells you either "Don't say that" or "It's alright to say that") is dysfunctional to some degree. Now you find yourself doing and saying things that were only thoughts before - thoughts you decided not to carry out.

When these types of things happen at home it is not good, but your family never says "You're fired" or "We are not in need of your services anymore." They may get irritated and disgusted, but usually you do not lose your job as husband, wife, daughter, or son. This, however, is not the case with employment. You can be in danger of losing your job if you "act before thinking."

Even though this behavior is a result of your brain injury, it does not mean that it is out of your control. You must take charge and bring your actions in check.

Examples

1. The work schedule is just posted and you see that the supervisor has scheduled you to work Saturday even though you told him you could not work that day. You immediately say, "What a jerk! Can't he ever get things right!" You turn around and see your boss face to face.

2. You insist that you cannot get the truck started, only to find that it's not in the right gear.

3. You get all upset when a shipment does not arrive that day. Upon later inspection you notice that it was supposed to arrive the next day.

4.	A group of co-workers are really yacking it up in the breakroom. You turn to your friend and say "How stupid."

5.	You get up and leave your company's staff meeting that goes overtime because you do not like to stay after quitting time.

6.	You blurt out "Who needs this job?"

7.	You perform your factory job in a careless manner without looking over your product.

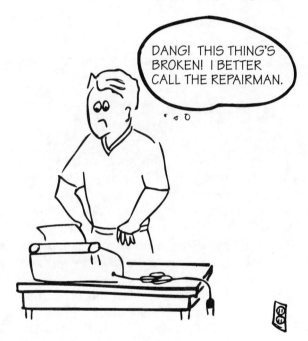

Compensation Techniques

1.	Try to develop a plan for counting to ten (10) before you act on anything.

2.	Always double-check your perception of a situation with a co-worker before you go off and act upon your understanding of the event.

3. Ask a trusted co-worker to tell you when he thinks you show impulsive actions.

4. Ask for more time on a project if you find yourself having to make snap decisions.

5. Go back over your actions at the end of the day. See if you can determine if there are behaviors you should control better next time around.

6. Slow down. Concentrate on everything you say or do.

7. Censor your conversations with your boss until this comes under more automatic control.

H. GETTING THINGS IN THE RIGHT ORDER

Have you been asked to complete a task at work and you find yourself confused as to where to start? This difficulty often leads to inertia or seeming lack of initiation as we discussed earlier. It can also lead to activities being completed out of order and, possibly, result in an inaccurate or incomplete job. Even though you may be trying your best, sequencing problems such as this can look like you are being careless, lazy, or just plain obstinate. Instead, you are confused or disoriented and will need to obtain assistance to learn tasks that require order to the automatic level - that is to say, second nature. There are a number of different approaches to overcoming this deficit, but the method is dependent upon the cause. It can be due to a variety or combination of deficits including comprehension, visual-spatial organization, visual synthesis and analysis, visual sequencing, or memory. Therefore, compensation techniques that you see on the job will be partially dependent upon the cause of the ordering problem.

Examples

1. You go to do a tune-up on a truck and find that you forgot to replace the plugs.

2. You start timing the hair permanent solution before you put it over the permanent rollers.

3. You mail over 100 envelopes, but do not include the letter dictated by your boss.

4. You find yourself confused about installing vinyl floor covering with a subfloor. It was second nature to you before.

5. You have forgotten certain procedures needed to perform your job as an accountant.

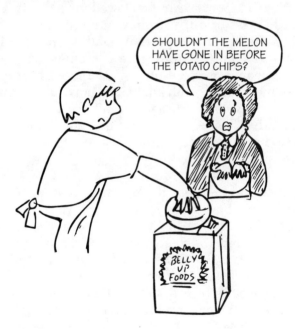

Compensation Techniques

1. Write down the correct steps to a task and refer back to your "cheat sheet" when necessary.

2. Have a co-worker or supervisor walk you through a task for practice.

3. Watch other people carefully when they are performing a task you find confusing.

4. Try to commit a sequence to memory using all the compensation strategies for visual memory. Talk yourself through it or visualize it for practice.

5. Always double-check your job activities for proper order and accuracy.

I. PERFORMING SLOWER THAN EXPECTED

Your responses can be slowed for a number of reasons. First of all, you may actually have gross or fine motor problems that lead to performing many tasks at a slower rate. Secondly, this delayed response may be due to decreased cognitive processing. Ideas and thoughts may take much longer to develop and, as a result, you do not act as quickly. Third, you may become easily distracted by other activities going on around your work space.

It would be great if jobs were only dependent on quality - how well you perform your finished product. But, the reality is that quantity is an important factor. In some jobs you can just work longer and get the same result. Unfortunately, in other types of employment you are required to meet a quota within a specified time and you are not allowed to work overtime to reach the goal.

Examples

1. You are required to sort 20 baskets of mail in a specified time. No matter how fast you try to go you cannot meet the basic criteria.

2. You are a receptionist who used to be able to handle irate customers with ease. Now you cannot think quickly enough of the best things to say.

3. Your typing speed is now only 30 words per minute.

4. When you come into the office on the week-end you can get two days work completed, but during weekdays you have great difficulty processing reports with other people in your work area.

5. Your day's activities do not get started until 10:00 AM because it takes you from 8:30 to 10:00 to get organized.

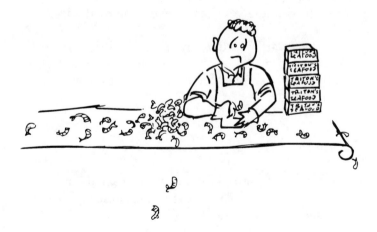

Compensation Techniques

1. Find a job that allows you to work overtime (without pay) in order to bring your production in line with minimum standards.

2. Practice tasks to the automatic level so you do not have to waste time thinking about what you must do.

3. If possible, look for a job that focuses on quality vs. quantity.

4. Look for a flexible boss.

J. BEING INFLEXIBLE

Oftentimes brain injury will result in rigidity and inflexibility. There are two ways to do things - yours, and the right way, and those two are synonymous. This thinking is sometimes due to a pre-morbid (pre-injury) personality trait, but can also be the result of concrete or "one-way" thinking. Because of cognitive deficits you have difficulty conceptualizing or visualizing a solution that is different from the one you have developed or devised.

Being able to look at multiple sides of an issue or to do a task more than one way is a sign of intelligence - so open your mind up to a variety of alternatives.

Examples

1. You find yourself arguing a great deal on the job over a disagreement on philosophical issues.

2. You do not want to change your shift even if it means a promotion with more money be-

cause you are used to the people on your current shift.

3. You have difficulty turning some activities over to a computerized system.

4. You are constantly upset that your boss is not there at 8:00 a.m. when you arrive, yet it does not concern you that he is at work until after dinner when you have gone home at 5:00 p.m.

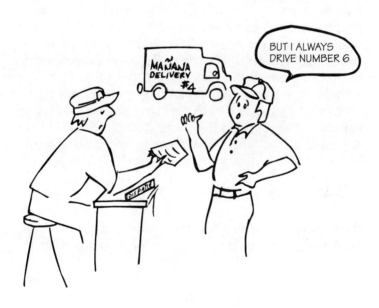

Compensation Techniques

1. Remember that there are often 20 effective ways of doing a task - your way is not the only one.

2. Try to view an idea from the other person's perspective.

3. Force yourself to do things differently, even if it is not required.

4. It is acceptable to ask why, but not acceptable to insist the explanation is wrong.

5. Try to minimize your stress on the job so that you can stay open to new thoughts and ideas.

K. ACTING DISORGANIZED

Possibly one of the first things that you realized was somewhat different after your injury was that you felt "spaced out," "disoriented", or "out of touch." Often times people with brain injury have these feelings remain with them over an extended period of time. What lingers is a problem defining a task, organizing the steps, and approaching each step in an organized fashion. You may be perfectly capable of accomplishing each step by itself, but a problem arises when you have to organize a total plan.

This may be a very difficult deficit for you to truly recognize in yourself. It is so easy to insist that "it is just a matter of opinion" and that your way is just as efficient as the other way that is being presented. We do not want to say that you will always be wrong; however, it is best to defer to others if they feel strongly that a different plan should be followed. Once you have been on the job for an extended period of time you can start to mildly challenge criticism of your approach.

Examples

1. You find yourself jumping from one job task to the next with no organized plan for your job activities that day.

2. You have difficulty prioritizing your job tasks.

3. You find it extremely frustrating that you cannot find a file that you are certain you were looking through just prior to going home the day before.

4. You are constantly late turning in reports to the boss.

5. You become confused easily when you try to reconstruct what you did the day before - mainly because you approached your tasks yesterday in such a haphazard manner.

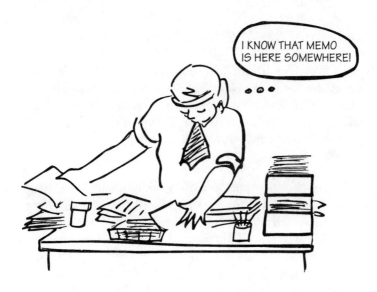

Compensation Techniques

1. Plan your activities for the week and keep reprioritizing on an as-needed basis.

2. Each morning make a list of things to accomplish for the day.

3. When you determine what projects you will address first, go over your plan with your supervisor.

4. Ask a trusted co-worker to let you know if he sees you struggling to present a "together appearance." Maybe he can give you some pointers.

5. Accept, accept, accept. If your boss says there is a better way to approach a project or task you should listen and try to comply. Even if you do not believe it is better, there is probably some reason for recommending the change. Besides that, the boss is always right.

L. SOLVING PROBLEMS

When you run into a problem on the job, you must be able to look at the issue, consider a number of ways to tackle the problem, and then choose a workable solution. After brain injury this process can break down at any one of these three steps.

In the first step you may experience confusion about what the problem really is, or you may even have difficulty recognizing that it is actually a problem area. This occurs because of thinking deficiencies discussed in the previous sections, such as remembering the problem exists, perceiving the issue correctly, comprehending what others have said, and understanding a sequence of events.

Secondly, you may have difficulty considering various methods of solving the problem. As we have described earlier, you may be fairly concrete or one-sided in how you look at the situation. In fact, you may only be able to "think" of one way to do it, so, naturally, that is what you try to suggest to others.

Lastly, you may be able to delineate some alternative solutions, yet not be able to choose the best one. They may all appear to be equally sound, or they may all have many drawbacks, that you cannot make a decision.

Examples

1. Mrs. Jones is on the telephone. She is irate that her carpet cannot be installed on the day you promised.

2. Your boss has asked you why you have not completed a project. Your part is finished, but your co-worker has not been able to do everything he needed to do. Your co-worker has asked you not to reveal this to the boss.

3. Every Friday you have to write up the work schedule for everybody in the grocery store. Many people have conflicting requests and no one says they can work on Christmas Day.

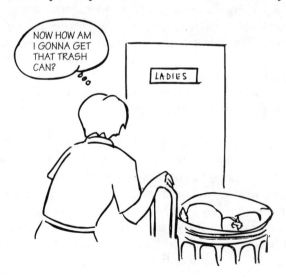

Compensation Techniques

1. When a problem arises, ask for clarification if you find yourself confused about the issues.

2. Never go for the first solution that comes into your head without attempting to consider alternatives.

3. Write out the possible solutions on paper and list the pros and cons to each.

4. If you have an understanding boss who is willing to give you a few minutes, ask him/her to check your decision. Be sure you go in prepared (alternatives laid out) and use a minimum of words to discuss your thoughts.

5. Do not let yourself get swayed by a verbal co-worker who is trying to coerce you into agreeing with him.

M. LEARNING NEW ACTIVITIES

After brain injury, old information is usually intact while new learning may be more difficult to master. This typically occurs when you have trouble taking in, either auditorially or visually, new data or facts. If you are familiar with at least part or parts of the job task, you will be better able to process the new aspects.

We are sure you can see that this has significant implications for job choices. In essence, your old job is going to be the one with which you will not encounter as many new learning demands. However, we are well aware that your "old job" may not be an alternative for a number of reasons including: physical limitations, uncooperative employer, or cognitive deficits.

The second best consideration would be a job that requires a large number of the skills you had to use in your former employment so that you can, at least, experience familiarity with parts of the environment. Again, we realize that the only alternatives may be something entirely different from your past skills. When this occurs you must be ready to experience some frustration with new learning, as well as the reality that preparing for a new career may take considerable time.

Examples

1. You used to be able to pick up new procedures on the job by watching someone do it only once.

2. You do not have any problems doing the projects that existed prior to your injury, but new projects are more difficult to grasp.

3. You find yourself talking excessively about a new account to everyone who will listen, but you are still not able to completely grasp all the issues.

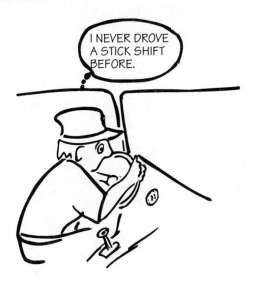

4.   You are still able to fix older model cars with ease, but the later ones with the newest technology are more time consuming.

Compensation Techniques

1.   Although it is often exciting to look at new job tasks, it will be more comfortable if you can initially return to work that is somewhat familiar.

2.   Remember that you may have to take more time to learn new activities - do not get discouraged.

3.   Be willing to work unpaid overtime to master new or different tasks.

4.   Try to break down the job into smaller parts so that you can master it efficiently.

5.   Do not be afraid to ask for additional help or a repeat of the instructions.

III. FEELING AND ACTING ON THE JOB

Returning to work is a major milestone in your rehabilitation. It will provide you with many benefits aside from money. Successful work re-entry can strengthen your sense of who you are and elevate your sense of self-worth. Successful work re-entry can provide you with a social network of friends and opportunities for closeness to others. Successful work re-entry can provide your life with a routine and purpose. Successful work re-entry can provide you with a sense of accomplishment. And, yes, believe it or not, your work can provide you with feelings of satisfaction and enjoyment. So, in addition to money, successful work re-entry can lead to a stronger sense of identity, increased self-esteem, greater intimacy, more meaning and direction, more enjoyment, and increased life satisfaction. All of this adds up to a better quality of life than you had experienced during your recovery and rehabilitation. We think you will agree with us that these benefits are worth the effort you will need to expend to obtain them.

Successful work re-entry just doesn't happen. You cannot sit back and wait for time to pass, nor can you expect others to make your return to work a big success. You cannot put yourself into "cruise" after you have found a job and expect to work happily ever after. No, sir! No, ma'am! You have to work at becoming a success on the job. Perhaps you have already arranged to adapt your work environment in consideration of any residual physical handicaps you possess. And maybe you have selected some of the compensatory techniques for cognitive deficits described in the last section of this manual. These adaptive and compensatory efforts are necessary and admirable, but they are not enough. In addition to these efforts, successful work re-entry depends upon how you control your feelings and actions. In fact, research has shown that the most frequent causes of the injured person's failure to return-to-work and on the job are unrestrained emotional and behavioral problems. If you want, therefore, to avoid failure and be a success on the job you must learn and practice ways to manage any residual emotional and/or behavioral problems you may have.

This section of the manual describes some of the residual, emotional, and behavioral problems after a brain injury. It will explore possible impacts these problems may have during your work re-entry. Lastly, it will suggest several ways you can deal with these problems. The objectives of this section are to help you:

1. Identify what emotional and behavioral problems you may still possess.

2. Recognize how these problems may affect your job performance.

3. Learn ways to better manage these problems.

The overall goal of this section, like other sections of the manual, is to facilitate your successful return-to-work.

The format for this section will be as follows: Symptoms, Causes, Job Impact, Solutions, and Action Plan. The *Symptoms* subsection describes the typical symptoms characteristic of each type of problem. The *Causes* subsection explains possible causes of the problem. The *Job Impact* subsection describes the possible effects the problem may have upon your job performance. The *Solutions* subsection will suggest several alternatives or courses of action that may help you better manage your problem. And the *Action Plan* subsection contains space for you to write down the course of action you intend to pursue to resolve or manage the problem.

The first step in solving almost any problem is identifying the existence and nature of the problem. This sounds easier than it is. Most of us prefer to ignore, avoid, minimize, rationalize or excuse our problems. Why? Because an awareness of them is, at least, uncomfortable and, at worst, mentally painful. Being basically pleasure seekers and pain avoiders, people have a tendency to either mentally or physically avoid their problems. You probably have this tendency, too. You will have to guard against this tendency if you want to identify the existence and nature of your problems. There are two important ingredients necessary to identify your problems: the desire to know them and the courage to face them. If you realize that problems that are denied or avoided remain and can even get worse and, if you recognize that problems can be opportunities for growth, then your desire to recognize and deal with them will increase. If you accept the fact that the problem-solving process is uncomfortable and, at times, painful but necessary, then you will realize you need to find the courage to see it through.

One of our clients asked us, "How do you know when you have a problem?" You may be wondering the same thing. Our response is that there are basically two ways to know when you have a problem: self-observation and feedback from others. You can identify your problem by observing your own thoughts, feelings, and actions. Another way you can identify your problems is feedback from others. This can be either oral or written feedback. Your family, friends, therapists, co-workers, and boss will give you feedback from time-to-time about some aspect of your behaviors. The feedback they give you can be a good source of information about your problems and difficulties. It is especially useful if several people are basically telling you the same thing. You should view this feedback as constructive criticism. You should welcome - and even invite - constructive feedback.

A third way to recognize whether or not you have a problem is provided in this manual. In each section detailing a social or emotional problem you will find a subsection entitled *Symptoms*. This subsection describes several possible symptoms characteristic of its respective problem. Scan this subsection. If you recognize a few symptoms judging from your self-observation or feedback from others, then there is a good chance you are presently experiencing or exhibiting that problem. Circle, underline, or highlight the symptoms you exhibit, then continue reading the other subsections.

After scanning the *Symptoms* subsection and recognizing they describe several symptoms you are currently experiencing, read the *Causes* subsection. The *Causes* subsection describes several possible causes of your problems and symptoms. Circle, underline, or highlight any causes you believe contribute to your problems and symptoms. It is important to identify possible causes of your problem and symptoms because they have a bearing on the solutions you will select and/or develop.

The next subsection is *Job Impact*. This subsection describes the impact your problems and symptoms will most likely have upon your job performance. The purpose of this subsection is to help you realize the effects and consequences your problem and symptoms can have upon your work. Hopefully, this awareness will motivate you to select and implement one or more solutions to your problem.

The subsection following *Job Impact* is *Solutions*. The *Solutions* subsection offers a variety of possible solutions to your problem. Circle, underline, or highlight a few that are appropriate for you.

The last subsection is entitled *Action Plan*. Once you have selected or developed solutions to your problem, you need to write out a plan about how and when you are going to implement these solutions. It is helpful to prioritize your solutions. The solutions whose outcomes are the most desirable and whose chances of being effective are high should be the highest in priority. Solutions high in priority should be given the most time, effort, and follow through.

So there you have it: a problem solving approach to the social-emotional problems that could hinder your successful return-to-work. Keep in mind the many benefits you stand to gain if your return-to-work is successful. Let these benefits provide you with the incentives to roll-up your sleeves and get to work on the social-emotional problems that might deny you these benefits. Good luck!

To facilitate your review and use of this section, "Feeling and Acting on the Job", the segments are arranged in the following order:

Symptoms

Causes

Job Impact

Solutions

Action Plan

Pay particular attention to the Action Plan. It will be most useful on your road to successful job re-entry.

A. ACCEPTING MY DEFICITS

Symptoms

The general problem that survivors of a brain injury often exhibit in this area is denial of deficits. What are some of the symptoms that might indicate you are not accepting some deficits? First, do you become overly hurt, upset, defensive, or hostile when others try to tell you of a weakness or deficit? Second, do you frequently discount, reject, or deny the validity of the constructive criticism others give to you? If you answered yes to one of these questions, chances are you currently experience the problem of "denial of deficits" to some degree. Some examples of this problem might help you better understand and recognize it. For example, you assert you are capable of driving a car when your doctor, therapists, family members, and friends tell you otherwise. Another example: you attribute the difficulty you are experiencing assembling something at work to a lack of glasses and not to the residual perceptual-motor deficits you have. You strongly insist that your memory difficulties are not significant and will not interfere with your vocational training or work performance. These are just a few examples to give you an understanding of this problem and, hopefully, help you recognize it more easily.

Causes

There are several possible causes of denial after a brain injury. One possible cause is organic - physical damage to a certain part of your brain that may have reduced your ability to perceive and monitor your physical, behavioral, cognitive, and emotional functioning. Another possible cause is psychological. Not only was your body traumatized by your injury, but your ego - psychological self was traumatized also. Consequently, it may be very weak and insecure. When the ego is weak and insecure it uses defense mechanisms to protect itself from perceived threats or dangers. Denial is one of the most common defense mechanisms used to protect the ego. When others give you constructive criticisms your ego perceives danger and reflexively resorts to denial to defend itself. Another possible cause could be lack of insight due to lack of feedback from others. We have observed that, sometimes after a brain injury, well-meaning friends and relatives withhold constructive feedback from the person with a brain injury. They rationalize that he cannot handle it or he is entitled to a few difficulties. Consequently, they let many difficulties, problems, or deficits "slide by" without confronting the person with these, silently saying to themselves, "He has had a brain injury, leave it alone." Lastly, difficulty acknowledging and accepting difficulties, deficits, and problems is a common human tendency as discussed in the introduction to this section. A brain injury exaggerates or magnifies this tendency to the point that it can cause significant problems.

Impact On Job

Denial of deficits can have a strong negative impact upon your work re-entry and job performance. For instance, whenever we attempt something new we are bound to make mistakes and need feedback from the environment and others to help us adapt. A person who denies their mistakes and rejects feedback will not adequently learn, nor adapt to new situations. Likewise, the person with a brain injury who denies his job errors and/or rejects feedback from his co-workers and employer will not adequently learn, nor adapt to his job. Another problem caused by denial of deficits is an unrealistic self-concept. The person with a brain injury harbors inaccurate, unrealistic beliefs about his capabilities. Consequently, he may make inappropriate vocational decisions or attempt inappropriate vocational tasks leading to high job stress, poor job performance, or even job failure (i.e., termination). Denial of deficits can also cause problems in your relations with your co-workers and employers. They may feel frustrated when you frequently deny your mistakes or reject their feedback. Eventually, they may give up trying to help you and even withdraw from you if you continue to deny your deficits. So denial of deficits can have an adverse affect upon your vocational decisions, adapting to and learning a new job, job performance, job stress, and relations with co-workers and employer. And, if these effects are not sufficient to motivate you to do something about your denial, here is another: denial of deficits can be the major obstacle to solving many of the problems in your life - social, emotional, cognitive, and vocational. So, as they say in the army, "It's a good place to start." Overcome your denial of deficits and you have done at least 50% of the hard work in learning to manage these problems.

Solutions

Below is a list of several possible solutions to help you overcome your tendency to deny your deficits and begin accepting them. Read them over. Mark the solutions you judge to be the most appropriate for your problem and the most likely to help you overcome this tendency.

1. Recognize that your tendency to deny your deficits is not due to stupidity, craziness, or dishonesty. Review the causes of denial and attempt to identify the cause of your denial. Use this insight to be compassionate with yourself when you recognize yourself denying your deficits. This will help you be less over-

whelmed by it, more likely to face it, and more likely to do something about it.

2. Cultivate a desire to have an accurate knowledge about yourself - strengths and weaknesses. Recognize that exercising the courage to face your "dark" side will help you grow, mature, and adapt. Often when we face the "truth" about ourselves we find out it is not as horrible as we had imagined. We find we are still worthy and lovable.

3. Ask someone you trust or feel close to - a trusted co-worker, your spouse, or a close friend - to tell you their perceptions of the difficulties you may be having.

4. When receiving constructive feedback, try not to be defensive, hurt, or hostile. Keep yourself calm by taking a few deep breaths, talking in a low voice, sitting down, and/or mentally counting backwards by 3s. After the person has given you the feedback do not counter with excuses, justifications, or rationalizations; instead, say back to the other person in your own words what you think you heard him/her say. After you have clarified the problem or deficit, ask the other person for more details about it: "How often do I do this?" "What effects does this have on others?," and so on.

5. Keep in mind, other people will respect you when you make a sincere effort to know and deal with your deficits.

6. Obtain and read reports about you written by your therapists. Identify your strengths and limitations. Discuss the implications of these strengths and limitations for your job functioning with your family, friends, vocational counselor, therapists, etc.

7. At work, ask one person to help you recognize when you are not being realistic about a vocational decision or task. Perhaps you can establish a special word or signal between you and this person that would tell you that you are denying something.

8. Join a local brain injury support group. Contact your nearest rehabilitation center for information about their meeting times and places. Other people with brain injury will not pull any punches with you. They will tell you like it is. They will tell you straight, even when you may not want to hear it.

9. If this problem is severe for you, ask your physician for a referral for professional counseling.

Action plan

To overcome your tendency to deny your deficits and begin to accept them, you have to do more than read and understand. You have to make some kind of action. An action plan is a plan to do certain things in order to achieve a goal or solve a problem. In the space provided below, rank order the solutions you selected according to the desirability of their outcome and probability of success. Add any extra solutions you thought up on your own. Write down how you will implement these solutions. Add specific details to make the general solutions more relevant to your situation.

_____

_____

_____

_____

_____

_____

_____

Now that you have completed your action
plan, post this plan in a convenient location so
that you can refer to it on a daily basis. This will
cue your memory and help maintain your motivation to follow through.

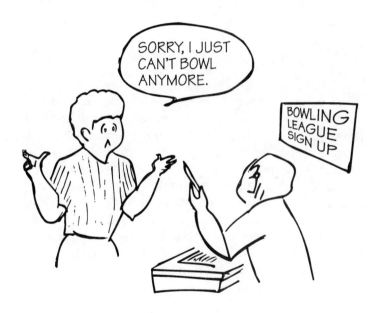

B. THINKING I CAN DO BETTER

Symptoms

A general problem you may be experiencing
is reduced or low self-esteem. You may believe that
you are not as competent or capable as you once
were. You may be feeling inadequate and even stupid. Consequently, with these beliefs and feelings

about yourself, you begin thinking you "can't cut it" or "can't do the job." What symptoms might you be experiencing or exhibiting that reflect this underlying problem? Feeling nervous or uptight on the job is one symptom. Dreading to go to work is another. Saying, "I can't," or "I don't know how" frequently is a third symptom. Expecting or waiting for others to do your job is another possible symptom. Putting yourself down by placing negative labels on yourself is also a symptom. Any one or a combination of these symptoms is a possible reflection of low self-esteem, feeling inadequate, and/or believing one is incompetent.

Causes

What are the causes of your low self-esteem after a brain injury? Changes in many aspects of yourself may be a major cause of your feelings of inadequacy and beliefs of incompetency. Changes in your appearance, motor skills, intellectual skills, emotional functioning, or personality can make you feel less competent compared to before your brain injury. Loss of occupation, reduced income, loss of status within the family, and loss of friends can make you feel less valuable, less worthy. Being unable to do the things you did before or, at least, not being able to do them as well can also contribute to feelings of inadequacy or beliefs of incompetency.

Impact on Job

Feeling inadequate or believing you are incapable can negatively affect your performance on the job in several ways. First, you experience more job stress and anxiety because you believe the work demands exceed your capabilities. Second, these feelings of inadequacy and thoughts of incompetency could lead to a "self-fulfilling" prophecy. In other words, you act *as if* you are inadequate or *as if* you are incompetent and, consequently, your job performance and productivity deteriorate, thereby fulfilling the negative prophecy you had about yourself. Third, you may be fearful to try something new or to advance in your career. Fourth, you may become overly dependent on your employer or co-workers for assistance with your job responsibilities. And fifth, as a result of the above, you may find yourself experiencing less enjoyment of the job and increased dissatisfaction with it.

Solutions

Below is a list of several things you can do to help yourself think you can do better and feel more adequate. Read them over and mark the solutions you believe are most appropriate for your situation and most probable for solving your problem.

1. It is important to explore and work through the many losses you sustained after a brain injury. But, it is also equally important to recognize the aspects of yourself that have not changed and the residual strengths you possess. Successful adaption after a brain injury often occurs via compensating for losses and limitations with remaining strengths in other areas. Learn what your strengths are and how you can use them to compensate for the challenges ahead of you. Inviting and receiving feedback from others about your strengths is one way to learn about them.

2. Remember that your job placement was most likely a decision based upon test data and the clinical judgments of one or more professionals. These persons would not knowingly place you in a position that you could not handle. Trust them and allow this trust to increase

your confidence in your potential to do your job.

3.   Remember also that often you are your own worst judge, your worst critic. Try to be more compassionate and patient with yourself. Talk back to your "critical self" when he/she is being unduly harsh or impatient.

4.   Overcome your perfectionist tendency by decreasing unrealistic, unhealthy, or impossible expectations and demands about yourself. Allow yourself the right to make mistakes. Learn how to deal with mistakes when you make them.

5.   Dwell upon your past and recent successes. Dwell upon your strengths. Use the positive images, memories, and feelings as the raw materials for elevating motivation and belief in yourself.

6.   Replace your internal critic's voice with the voice of self-talk. Praise yourself when you do something well. Affirm yourself with statements about your worth, capabilities, and potential.

7.   Challenge the negative labels you place on yourself. Often they are extreme, exaggerated, or distorted. Ask upon what evidence they are based. Rebut the logic of the conclusion on which they are based. Substitute more precise language for them (e.g., Replace "I am a fat slob" with "I am x pounds overweight).

8.   Set realistic, attainable, short-term work goals. Write them down on paper. Write out an action plan for their attainment. Act upon the plan. Note your successes.

9. Cope, don't mope! Don't just complain about your problem(s). Take some action to remediate or compensate for the weakness or limitation.

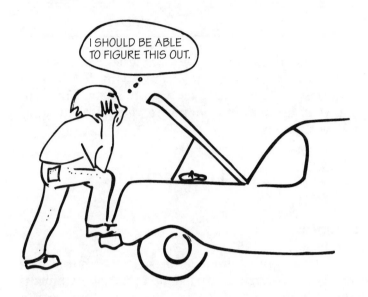

Action Plan

Now that you have recognized the symptoms of your problem, determined possible causes, and selected several solutions, the next step is to write out an "Action Plan" detailing the priority, means, and specifics of the solutions. Rank order the solutions you have selected according to the desirability of their outcome(s) and probability of success. Write down how you will implement the solution. Add specific details to make the general solution more relevent to a particular problem:

_____

_____

_____

_____

_____

_____

_____

Now that you have completed your action plan, post this plan in a convenient location so that you can refer to it on a daily basis. This will cue your memory and maintain your motivation to follow through.

C. FEELING GROUCHY

Symptoms

After a brain injury almost every injured person goes through a period of agitation. Unfortunately, for a significant number of persons with a brain injury, the problem never goes completely away. They remain grouchy or irritable for the rest of their lives. Do you have this problem? One way to recognize whether or not this is a problem for you is to survey its symptoms. The primary symptom is a negative mood akin to possessing a diffuse or nondirected anger. Your "fuse" seems much shorter than it was prior to your brain injury. You have less patience with people. You become more easily upset than you did in the past. Your tolerence for frustration is significantly reduced. You do not seem capable of selectively focusing your attention and concentrating on something for any significant length of time. You are more restless and edgy than before, especially when stress is moderate to high and/or sleep has been poor. Lastly, you may have noticed your conflicts with others are more frequent and severe.

Causes

Your increased irritability or grouchiness is primarily due to organic causes, and secondarily due to situational causes. Your brain injury resulted in organic damage to the brain that affected one or more important capabilities. Changes in your ability to accurately perceive and understand social situations can cause increased irritability. Difficulty in performing simple, routine tasks that used to be automatic for you can cause increased irritability. Problems filtering out extraneous noises in the environment can also cause increased irritability. Situational factors also play a secondary role in your irritability. Maybe you have noticed your level of irritability increases as the noise, demands and stress of your surroundings increase. Also, there are certain persons and groups of people who may trigger higher levels of irritability in you. For instance, adult persons with brain injuries tend to be more irritable around children and adolescents. Again, the primary cause of your irritability is organic, but situational factors can also be a contributing cause.

Impact on Job

Being grouchy or irritable can have a negative impact on your vocational life. Perhaps the most difficulty it will cause you is in the area of social relations on the job. When you are irritable you make the work environment unpleasant for your co-workers. Others are uncomfortable with you when you are frequently "out of sorts." If the frequency, duration, and/or intensity of your irritability is high, your co-workers will begin to avoid you. This avoidance by others could cause you to feel very lonely and isolated in the job setting. Irritability will also stand in the way of your job satisfaction and enjoyment. It is near to impossible to derive satisfaction or enjoyment from any activity when you are "out of sorts." So you see, irritability on the job can hurt your social relations with your co-workers and prevent you from experiencing job satisfaction and enjoyment.

Solutions

Below is a list of several possible solutions to help you cope with irritability. Read them over. Mark the solutions you judge to be the most appropriate for your problem and the most likely to meet with success in solving your problem.

1. Reduce the distractions and background noises in your work environment. Enlist the support of your employer and co-workers by asking them for suggestions on how to best do this.

2. Plan your day. Schedule difficult tasks when you are at your best, which is usually the morning hours for most persons with a brain injury.

3. Learn relaxation techniques and practice them twice a day for approximately 15 minutes per session. Buy a book and cassette tapes on relaxation techniques or take an evening class on them to help you learn and master these skills.

4. Explore and evaluate your expectations about yourself, others, and your job. Unrealistic, perfectionistic expectations predispose you to be continually angry and irritable. Replace these unhealthy expectations with more realistic, human expectations.

5. Learn assertive communication skills. Apply them on the job and you will increase the probability of getting what you want, improve

your relations with others, and, thereby, reduce your level of irritability.

6. Learn and practice good breathing techniques. Use breathing exercises at the onset of irritability to counter its escalation.

7. Use the power of your imagination to visualize ways of successfully handling difficult situations or persons in advance of the event itself.

8. Join a support group for persons with a brain injury. Discuss your irritability problem with the group. Use the group as a sounding-board and a source of potential suggestions for coping with this problem.

9. Ask your physician for recommendations about an exercise regimen you can follow to indirectly reduce your level of irritability.

10. If your irritability is severely impacting upon your functioning in the home or work setting, then ask your physician for a referral or professional counseling.

Action Plan

One of the primary causes of failure to attain a goal is failure to write it down. A second cause of failure in goal-seeking is lack of a plan. In the space below, rank order the solutions you have selected according to the desirability of their outcome and probability of success. Write down how you will implement the solution. Add specific details to make the general solution more relevant to your particular problem.

_____

_____

_____

_____

_____

_____

_____

Now that you have completed your action plan, post your plan in a convenient location so that you can refer to it on a daily basis. This will cue your memory and maintain your motivation to follow through.

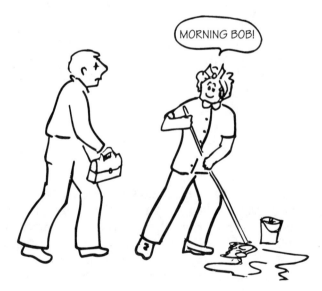

D. ACTING IMPATIENT

Symptoms

Many survivors of a brain injury are quite often impatient and it is most likely that you are no exception. Do you find yourself frequently frustrated or irritated with people or things because they don't seem to move fast enough? Do you find yourself frequently exasperated because others do not seem to see things the way you do or do not want to do things your way? Do you find it much more difficult to wait? Do you become irate if you have to wait more than 10 minutes? Do you have trouble tolerating others when they cannot understand what you have said and you have to explain it again? Frustration, irritation, exasperation, difficulty waiting, blowups, and intolerance are some of the symptoms of impatience. If you answered "yes" to any of the questions above, chances are this is one of your problems.

Causes

What are the causes of impatience after a brain injury? One cause may be organic. The part of your brain that regulates your emotions has been damaged, thus, your ability to control emotions, especially negative ones - has been reduced. Other possible causes are psychological. A brain injury often results in self-centeredness and difficulty seeing another's perspective. This deficit adversely affects your social interactions because being able to anticipate another's perspective and temporarily postpone our own helps us to be tolerant, understanding, and patient. Another psychological factor that could contribute to this problem is "racing thoughts." Some of our clients have told us that the thoughts in their mind seem to go much faster than before their brain injury. They maintain that this makes it difficult for them during conversations and social transactions. A third psychological cause of impatience after a brain injury is reduced frustration/stress tolerance. Clients report that they have to work so much harder to do everyday things that before their brain injury were automatic and effortless. Consequently, they experience more stress and are, therefore, more impatient than they would be if they were not so stressed. Lastly, a fact we must all acknowledge is that life after a brain injury is filled with more frustrations, disappointments, and hassles than life before the injury. Consequently, you reach your frustration, disappointment, and hassle "quota" faster than before and your patience runs out.

Impact on Job

You have heard the expression, "Haste makes waste;" that means going too fast can cause costly errors. This is one of the negative impacts of impatience upon your job performance. You try to do things too fast and end up making costly mistakes. This, in turn, reduces your productivity and decreases your competency. If you continue to act this way, you reduce your overall value as an employee and run the risk of losing your job. Another problem impatience creates on the job is pressure - on yourself and others. You feel a lot of internal pressure from all the negative emotions building up inside of you; your co-workers feel pressure because you are frequently telling them what to do, wanting them to do things your way, or becoming upset when things are not the way you want or think they should be. They begin to feel like they are "walking on eggshells" when you are around. This is very uncomfortable for them and may result in them avoiding you. Decreased productivity and strained relations with your co-workers will lead to an increase in job dissatisfaction which, in turn, may result in a desire to quit your job. Of course, quitting is not the answer; learning to reduce, control, or eliminate your impatience is (the answer).

Solutions

Below is a list of several possible solutions to help you reduce, control, or eliminate (temporarily) your impatience. Read them over. Mark the solutions you judge to be the most appropriate for your impatience and the most likely to help you manage it.

1. Remember that recovery from brain injury is a long process that requires both time and effort. Do not force it or terminate your therapies prematurely. Allow others to help you.

2. Identify the situations, tasks, and people that challenge your patience. Figure out, ahead of time, some ways of dealing with these situations, tasks, or people that would be less trying for you.

3. Recognize that your view of things or way of doing things is not the only way of viewing or doing things. Recognize that others' ways of viewing and doing things may be just as valid. Act upon this awareness by asking others how they view things and what they believe is a good way to do things.

4. Make sure you are getting adequate sleep and nutrition. Many of our clients report they need more sleep after having had a brain injury than before their injury. Being rested and properly nourished will increase your physical stamina and mental tolerance, thereby reducing your fatigue, irritability, and impatience.

5. Learn and practice relaxation techniques. It is generally recommended that one practice these techniques twice a day to lower their overall stress thermostat. Learn from books, cassette tapes, or workshops about the variety of relaxation techniques available. Find two that work for you.

6. On the job, take short breaks when appropriate.

7. On the job, use caution when setting task goals and time frames. Remember you will probably need more time and effort to complete tasks than before.

8. Learn to communicate your ideas to fellow coworkers in a respectful fashion, but also be willing to listen respectfully to their ideas.

9. When you need to blow off steam, select an appropriate time, place, and person. Do not indiscriminately dump your negative feelings of frustration, irritation, intolerance, exasperation, and impatience on innocent bystanders, or in an unproductive fashion or place.

10. Learn positive, realistic self-talk to regulate your impatience.

Action Plan

Impatience is a challenging emotion. You are going to have to diligently work at it if you want to successfully manage it. The first step is having a plan. In the space below, rank order the solutions that you have identified to this problem. Rank order the solutions by the desirability of their outcomes and the probability of their success for you. Write down how you will implement them. Be as specific as you can. Add any details that will tailor these general solutions to your specific problem.

_____

_____

_____

_____

_____

_____

_____

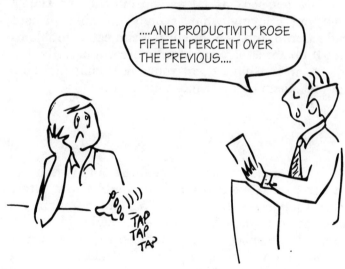

Now that you have completed your action plan, post your plan in a convenient location so that you can refer to it on a daily basis. This will cue your memory and maintain your motivation to follow through.

E. SPEAKING OUT

Symptoms

"Speaking out" means saying things that are insensitive, rude, hurtful, mean, or thoughtless. You say the first thing that pops into your head without censoring or editing. As a result, you often say aloud things you only would have thought, but not spoken in the past. For instance, if a prospective employer called to tell you he had decided to hire someone else, you might bluntly reply, "I didn't want to work at your stupid business anyway. You couldn't pay me enough." Another example: a friend of yours who is dieting comes over to your house for dinner. When she arrives you tactlessly state, "Boy, your diet must not be working because you look as fat as you did the last time I saw you." Saying what is on your mind without reflection, inhibition, or editing can cause problems in all domains of your life. Before we describe the effects it can have upon your vocational functioning, let's examine possible causes of it.

Causes

The major cause of "speaking out" is damage to the part of your brain that inhibits and filters your thoughts. This means that the mechanisms that govern the expression of thoughts are deficient. As a consequence, you often say whatever is on your mind. This is especially pronounced during times of emotional distress.

Impact on Job

Saying the first thought that pops into your mind, especially when the thought is cruel, mean, or hurtful, will quickly disrupt social relations on the job. Thoughtless comments can embarrass, offend, hurt, and anger your fellow co-workers. They may think of you as mean, cruel, insensitive, or peculiar. Once they form this negative impression of you and experience several uncomfortable transactions with you, they may write you off and decide that they do not want to associate with you. This, in turn, can lead to you becoming socially isolated on the job. This will reduce the amount of enjoyment and satisfaction you could have gained from your work.

Solutions

Below is a list of several possible solutions to help you manage and control your impulse to speak out. Read them over. Mark the solutions you judge to be the most appropriate for your problem, and the most likely to help you manage it.

1. Pause a few seconds before you speak. Never say anything immediately. Stop and listen to your thoughts before you speak them. Ask yourself, "Would this thought be constructive or destructive to this communication transaction or relationship?" Speak those thoughts that are constructive.

2. Compartmentalize this tendency by only making blunt, joking, or sarcastic remarks to a close friend and not making these types of remarks to others.

3. Talk with a friend about this problem. Ask your friend to describe several instances of your "speaking out" and the effects this had upon others. Ask your friend what types of comments would have been more appropriate.

4. On the job enlist the help of a trusted co-worker. Ask him or her to give you a signal or

sign when your communication is impulsive or inappropriate. When you get this sign or signal, stop talking, apologize, and change your communication to something more appropriate.

5. Before social interactions, decide ahead of time some general topics you wish to discuss. During social interactions silently talk to yourself in your mind's ear and direct your communication behaviors along these topics.

6. If this problem is severe and/or you cannot manage it on your own, request your physician to refer you to an appropriate professional for help with this.

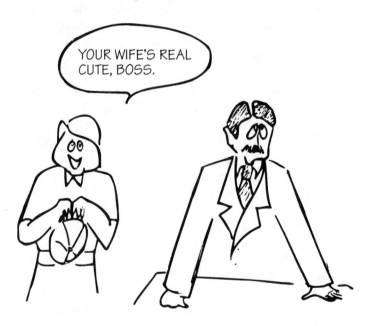

YOUR WIFE'S REAL CUTE, BOSS.

Action Plan

Controlling an impulse is tough. It requires hard work and diligence. You definitely have to have a plan of action and implement this plan on a daily basis if you really want to control an impulse. In the space provided below, rank order the solutions by the desirability of their outcome and probability of success for your problem. Add specific details to make the general solutions more relevant to your situation. Write down how you will implement your solutions.

_____

_____

_____

_____

_____

_____

_____

Now that you have completed your action plan, post your plan in a convenient location so that you can refer to it on a daily basis. This will cue your memory and maintain your motivation to follow through.

F. ACTING OUT

Symptoms

Acting out means physically expressing your anger or frustration in an impulsive (without thinking) fashion. It is often an overreaction to an unpleasant or stressful situation. A symptom of this problem is physical outbursts (i.e., throwing, hitting, tearing, breaking, kicking, etc.) that are excessive or out of proportion to the precipitating (triggering) situation.

Causes

The primary cause of your acting out is organic impairment of your filtering system. This means that areas of your brain that would normally inhibit such behaviors are dysfunctional. Consequently, your acting out is often an automatic or reflexive reaction to any form of frustration or stress. Hence, frustrating or stressful situations, persons, or objects are secondary or indirect causes of your acting out.

Impact on Job

Acting out or physical outbursts will have a severe and immediate impact on your job status. Because physical outbursts have the potential for harm and destruction, your employer and co-workers will have very little tolerance for this type of behavior. If you are not fired, you will not be respected nor liked very much by your employer and co-workers. Again, this will lead to social avoidance and rejection of you by others. This, in turn, will result in feelings of isolation and loneliness. Once again, this negative fall out will result in less job satisfaction and enjoyment.

Solutions

Below is a list of several possible solutions to help you cope with "acting out". Read them over. Mark the solutions you judge to be the most appropriate for your problem and the most likely to meet with success in solving it.

1. When you feel yourself becoming upset, stop, take several (3-5) even, rhythmic deep breaths. This will help calm down your bodily reactions. Next, silently count backwards in

your mind so as to distract it from the object of arousal and calm the mind.

2. Learn relaxation techniques and practice them twice a day for approximately 15 minutes per session. Buy a book and cassette tapes on relaxation techniques or take an evening class on it to help you learn and master these skills.

3. Try to identify, in advance, situations, events, persons, places, etc. that are frustrating, upsetting, and/or stressful for you. Mentally rehearse what you will say and how you will act at the beginning, middle, and end of the transaction. It might be helpful to initially write-out a script about what you would say or do.

4. After a physical outburst, apologize to others, make physical restitution if necessary, and explore how you could have handled it better.

5. When you feel anger building, force yourself to sit down and speak in a calm tone of voice.

6. When your anger begins to approach rage, tell the others present that you want to take a "time out." Then immediately leave the situation and engage yourself in some type of constructive activity.

7. Learn and practice assertive communication skills.

8. Before you get bent out of shape about something, remember these three words: "Check It Out!" Overreaction is frequently caused by misperceptions and misunderstandings. Before you fly off the handle, ask questions to get the facts straight.

9. Consult your physician for assistance with this problem. He may recommend drug therapy and/or psychological therapy.

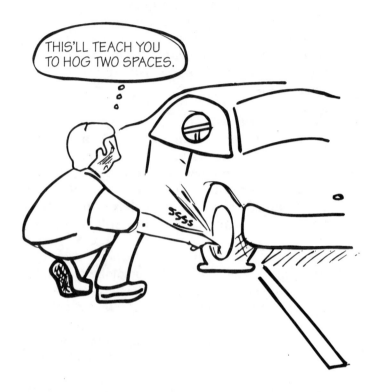

Action Plan

To go from the drawing board to real life you need a plan. Use the space below to develop a plan to manage your acting out behaviors. Rank order the solutions you selected above according to their appropriateness for your problem and the probability of success in solving it. Write down how you will implement your plan. Add specific details to make the general solution more relevant to your particular problem.

_____

_____

_____

_____

_____

_____

_____

Now that you have completed your action plan, post your plan in a convenient location so that you can refer to it on a daily basis. This will cue your memory and maintain your motivation to follow through.

G. ZEROING IN ON ME

Symptoms

It is natural for someone who has experienced a traumatic injury to focus primarily on himself. This is a built in psychological survival mechanism. When you suffered your trauma this happened to you. At first you were very self-centered. You focused entirely on yourself. Your ability to empathize with the thoughts and feelings of others was very low or nonexistent. Your perception of events around you were in terms of how they related to you. Most of your conversations revolved around your concerns, needs, plans, wants, and wishes. The problem we are describing is called "egocentricism". "Ego" means self, "centricism" means "centered." So by egocentricism we mean the problem of being excessively self-centered.

Presently you are not as egocentric as you were. You are probably more aware of others' thoughts, feelings, needs, and actions. Most likely you do things for others, too. Nonetheless, for some there is a residual amount of "egocentricism" that can still cause problems. Here are some questions to ask yourself to check if you may currently have some traces of this problem.

1. Are your thoughts often about yourself?

2. Are your conversations often focused on your concerns, needs, wants, plans, etc.?

3. Do you often experience jealousy when your spouse, friend, therapist interacts with another?

4. Do you often interrupt others to tell them your point of view or turn the conversation's focus onto yourself?

5. Do others accuse you of being selfish?

If you answered "yes" to two or more questions, chances are you are experiencing a residual amount of egocentricism that may be currently causing problems for you.

Causes

Egocentricism after a brain injury is caused by psychological, organic, and situational factors. As alluded to earlier, the physical trauma you suffered also traumatized your ego. Egocentricism is a typical, psychological reaction presumably arising from the ego's will to survive. Egocentricism is also maintained by damage to the brain, specifically the frontal lobes. You may have lost some of the intellectual capacity to assume or anticipate another's thoughts, feelings, and needs. Lastly, the nature of the rehabilitation process - both acute and chronic - may foster some egocentricism. During this lengthy process the time, efforts, and concerns of many persons are focused on you. This indirectly reinforces your egocentricism. Perhaps you remember experiencing some withdrawal pangs as your rehabilitation became less intensive and health professionals began to disengage from you. So there are three primary causes of egocentricism - psychological, organic, and situational. These primary causes can be supplemented by secondary ones such as your personality characteristics prior to your brain injury. Generally speaking, if you had a tendency to be self-centered before your injury, this tendency is often magnified after a brain injury.

Impact on Job

Being too egocentric can have an adverse effect upon your job functioning. Socially, you may have difficulty engaging in small talk or the give and take of conversation; consequently you may fail to develop any significant relations with co-workers. Others may perceive you as selfish or self-centered and not seek to associate with you nor form a friendship. If you continue to only think of yourself and ignore the concerns and needs of others, they may begin to think of you as being inconsiderate or uncaring. Egocentricism can also affect your job performance. You may have difficulty perceiving others' views on how to do a job. You may insist on doing things "my way." You may become upset if things are not done your way. All of this can cause friction between co-workers and tension on the job.

Solutions

Below is a list of possible solutions that may help you decenter and focus more on the thoughts, feelings, needs, views, and concerns of others.

Read them over. Mark the solutions you judge to be appropriate for your problem and the ones most likely to help solve it.

1. Ask someone you trust (i.e., spouse, therapist, good friend) if you have an "I" problem. In other words, ask, "Do I talk about myself too much?" "Do you think I listen well to others?," "Am I concerned with others' thoughts, feelings, and needs?"

2. Ask this trusted person to signal you or give you feedback when your conversations or actions are too self-centered.

3. Recognize that a world inhabited by one person is a very small world indeed! Expand your world and universe by looking outward to others. Ask them how they are doing and really listen. Follow up this question with more questions about their thoughts, feelings, experiences, concerns, opinions, etc. Not only will your world expand, but soon you will find it inhabited by friends and acquaintances.

4. Count the number of "I's" in your conversations. If there are too many, decrease them and substitute "you" and ask questions about others in their place.

5. Look for ways to help someone else instead of expecting them to help you. Helping others can be very gratifying and uplifting.

6. Become involved in a brain injury support group or volunteer organization. These groups will give you opportunities to help others.

7. Be discriminating in picking the times, places, and persons for indulging in conversations about your thoughts, feelings, concerns, needs, wishes, wants, goals, etc. Set a time

limit for these sessions. And do not ignore the thoughts, feelings, concerns, and needs of the person with whom you are interacting.

8.   If your egocentricism is moderate to severe and you are unable to manage it on your own after trying, ask your physician for a referral for professional assistance with the problem.

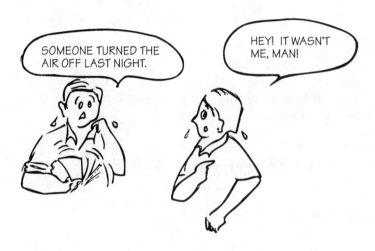

Action Plan

Decentering and focusing on others requires time, effort, and strategies. An action plan can map out the strategies you will use to accomplish these objectives. Take the time to develop your personal plan. Use the space below to rank order the solutions you selected above. Rank order them according to their appropriateness for your problem and probability of success in solving it. Add specific details to tailor the general solutions to your situation.

_____

_____

_____

_____

_____

_____

Now that you have completed your action plan, post your plan in a convenient location so that you can refer to it on a daily basis. This will cue your memory and maintain your motivation to follow through.

H. OVERWHELMED BY EMOTION

Symptoms

The general problem in this area is called "lability." Lability describes a loss of control over one's emotional reactions. This may be manifested by crying more often or more intensely, laughing too much or at inappropriate times, experiencing rage reactions or anxiety attacks. All of these emotional reactions are often an overreaction to the event that precipitated them. These overreactions have, most likely, been embarrassing experiences for you.

Causes

The primary cause of being overwhelmed by emotions (lability) is organic. The areas of your brain that handle your emotions have been affected by your injury. Consequently, your emotions seem to be closer to the surface and quickly arise when you face stressful or emotionally laden events. A secondary cause of emotional overreactions is social misperception or misunderstanding. Sometimes you may not accurately perceive or understand the social information around you. With the passage of time you may have noticed that you have regained some emotional control; however, you will probably never attain the same degree of control you had prior to your injury.

Impact on Job

The impact emotional lability will have upon your job performance will vary depending upon its nature (what emotion?), frequency (how often?), intensity (how severe?), and duration (how long?). Generally, the more frequent, intense, and longer lasting emotions will be more disruptive to your work than emotions that are less frequent, less intense, and of shorter duration. Anger and rage have a more severe impact than anxiety or excessive laughter. The least serious effect is embarrassment within yourself and mild discomfort in others. The more serious effects are anger, hostility, and high stress in the work place.

Solutions

Below is a list of possible solutions that may help you regain more control of your emotions or, at least, reduce the frequency, intensity, or duration of emotionally labile episodes. Read them over. Mark the solutions that are appropriate for your problem and the most likely to help you solve it.

1. Be aware of your limitations. Use this knowledge to make sound decisions about jobs,

tasks, and people you can cope with, and identify those you cannot. Avoid activities, jobs, tasks, or persons you cannot honestly deal with or, at least, get assistance and support to help you if you must deal with challenges that are beyond your limitations.

2. Learn and practice daily relaxation techniques. Practicing relaxation techniques will help reduce the frequency, intensity, and duration of your states of tension and increase the frequency, intensity, and duration of states of relaxation. Relaxation states inhibit the emergency nervous system (sympathetic nervous system) and trigger the resting nervous system (parasympathetic nervous system). The overall result is a better, more relaxed mood - one more resistive to stress and less prone to overreaction.

3. Sometimes your emotional overreaction is due to social misperception or misunderstanding. You can reduce the frequency, intensity, and duration of some of your emotional reactions by correcting your misperception and misunderstanding. We often advise our clients to "Check It Out" before jumping to conclusions and emotionally reacting. This means to postpone your conclusions and reactions to an event until after you have an accurate, clear picture of it. This often requires asking questions of another and paraphrasing back your perceptions and understanding until your perceptions and understanding are accurate. It only takes an extra few minutes, but the payoffs are well worth it.

4. Using positive, realistic self-talk before, during, and after emotional over reactions can help better manage them and reduce their frequency, intensity, and duration in the future. Positive self-talk is an internal dialogue

with yourself in your head. Of course, you can speak aloud to yourself if you are alone and it would not be socially inappropriate. During realistic, positive self-talk you tell yourself a realistic appraisal of the event you are experiencing and a positive expectation of your capacity to deal with it. For instance, if you are facing an imminent job interview you might say, "OK, Jack, you're nervous about this interview. That's understandable, but, remember, it's not the last job interview in the world. If it doesn't turn out there are other jobs. Besides, you're prepared. You're dressed for success; you've rehearsed for the interview; and you know you can do the job if given a chance. So give it your best shot - that's all anyone can do - and let the chips fall where they may." This type of self-talk in this situation may lower the intensity of anxiety to a more manageable level and bolster self-confidence a few degrees. The net result is a slightly higher degree of emotional control producing a possible significant difference between social catastrophe and social functioning.

5. If your emotional lability is moderate to severe and you are unable to manage it on your own after some effort, consult with your physician about it. He may prescribe some type of temporary drug therapy and/or refer you for psychotherapy for this problem.

Action Plan

Regaining control of your emotions is a very important and challenging task. It is necessary for your social-emotional adjustment in both work and home environments. A plan of action on how you will regain and increase your emotional control is essential. In the space below, write out the solutions you marked above. Rank order them by the desirability of their outcome and the probability of success for your problem. Add specific details to make the general solutions more relevant to your situation. Write down how you will implement your solutions.

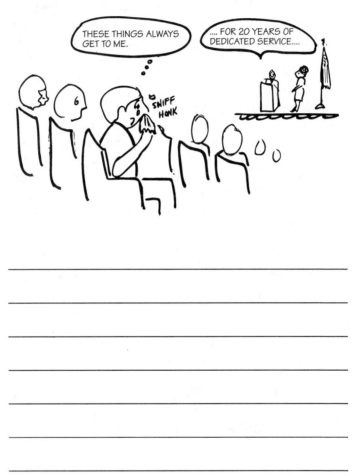

Now that you have completed your action plan, post your plan in a convenient location so that you can refer to it on a daily basis. This will cue your memory and maintain your motivation to follow through.

I. OVERCOMING DEPRESSION

Symptoms

Depression is a mood disorder that contains numerous thinking, feeling, and acting symptoms. The onset of depression occurs when your perception of the reality of your losses becomes more accurate. When you perceive this reality you experience numerous negative emotions: extreme sadness, a deep sense of loss, hopelessness, helplessness, loss of enjoyment. Your motivation is also affected. Your initiative decreases, apathy increases, and your overall energy and motivation decline. Your thought processes are also adversely affected. Your thinking becomes negativistic, pessimistic, distorted, and irrational. Not only are your thoughts about the present and future blackened, but your memories of the past are invaded by your depression, much like a computer virus ravages the memory storage of a computer. Depression can insidiously cause your bright memories of the past to be rewritten in a black, negative tone - disregarding the good and exaggerating the bad. Depression also has a negative impact upon your behavior. Staying in bed until the afternoon, inactivity, watching television for countless hours, and suicidal attempts are some of the behavioral manifestations of depression. Many persons have descibed depression as like being in a dark psychological prison.

Causes

Depression after a brain injury has many causes. The primary cause is often organic. Damage to certain brain structures or a change in the brain chemistry (i.e., neurotransmitters) can cause depression. The many losses one must confront and cope with after a brain injury are another major cause of depression. Loss of identity, body image, occupation, income, status, power control, skills, etc. are some of these losses. Depression can also arise from the chronic stress and burnout one may experience during the long recovery and rehabilitation process after a brain injury. These are the major, but not the only, causes of depression after a brain injury.

Impact on Job

Looking over the many significant symptoms of depression, you will quickly realize that it has an adverse effect upon job functioning. Apathy, lack of motivation, and lack of initiative make it extremely difficult to find the energy or incentive to perform. The heavy, negative mood of depression is a downer to co-workers. They also feel perplexed and frustrated when their attempts to console and assist you are unsuccessful. Your employer is also concerned. On the one hand, he is probably concerned about your mental health and, on the other, he is concerned about your job performance. Next to the poor anger control, coping with depression is a challenging problem for everyone involved.

Solutions

Below is a list of several possible solutions to help you manage your depression. Read them over. Mark the solutions you judge to be the most appropriate for your problem and the most likely to meet with success in solving it.

1.   Consult with your doctor about the possibility of organic factors contributing to your depression. If this is so, he may prescribe some form of drug therapy.

2. Educate yourself about the nature and cause of depression and techniques for its management. Your local library or bookstore should have books and cassettes on this topic.

3. Diagnose the nature and severity of your depression using questionnaires provided in the books cited above. If your depression is in the moderate to severe range you should seek counseling.

4. Begin keeping a daily - or at least weekly -record of your mood. Review self-help books for form or information.

5. Learn about the relationship between your thoughts and your mood. Recognize the role negative or distorted thoughts play in negative emotions. Learn how you can control your mood by correcting your thought distortions.

6. Make a point to always look your best. Decide ahead of time about your grooming and appearance.

7. Make an effort to plan out your day the night before or in the early morning hours.

8. Obtain training in social skills and relaxation techniques. Research has shown that these skills can have an indirect positive effect on depression.

9. Become involved in a support group. Establish a buddy system with a member of the group who is coping with the same problem. Share ideas on coping. Encourage one another in your efforts.

Action Plan

If you want to go somewhere - especially someplace unfamiliar to you - it helps to use a map. Likewise, when you want to overcome a problem and grow, it helps to have an action plan. Use the space below to develop your action plan to manage your depression. Rank order the solutions you selected above according to their appropriateness for your problem and their probability of success in solving it. Write down how you will implement your plan. Add specific details to make the general solutions more relevant to your particular problem.

_____

_____

_____

_____

_____

_____

Now that you have completed your action plan, post your plan in a convenient location so that you can refer to it on a daily basis. This will cue your memory and maintain your motivation to follow through.

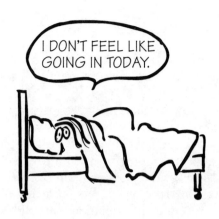

J. EXPERIENCING A LACK OF MOTIVATION

Symptoms

Has your "get up and go" got up and went? Do you feel like nothing is of any real importance? Have you stopped caring about things? Do you feel like not doing a thing? Are you frequently procrastinating in your work and home responsibilities? Are you spending most of your non-working hours watching television? Have you lost interest in your previous hobbies? Have you stopped experiencing the feeling of enjoyment? If you answered "yes" to any of the questions above, chances are you are experiencing a lack of motivation to some degree. Your lack of motivation can range from mild, such as procrastinating in everyday work and home responsibilities, to extreme, such as total do-nothingness when you don't want to get out of bed.

Causes

Initially, right after your brain injury, your lack of motivation was primarily due to an organic factor. The parts of your brain that energize and direct your behavior were dysfunctional. Your drive was reduced; your fatigue was increased. You were confused and had difficulty conceptualizing, planning, and following through with activities. All projects or goals, however small, were overwhelming. As you recovered, the severity of this type of lack of motivation subsided, but did not disappear entirely. A certain amount of lack of motivation remained in the form of lack of initiative, lack of movement, or inertia. As time passes, the organic cause of your lack of motivation diminishes and is surpassed by psychological causes: depression and negative mind-sets. Depression can paralyze your willpower and trap you in emotional prison for weeks, months, and even years. There are numerous negative mind-sets that can also cause a lack of motivation: hopelessness, helplessness, overwhelming yourself, jumping to conclusions, self-labeling, undervaluing rewards, perfectionism, fear of failure, fear of success, fear of disapproval or criticism, coercion and resentment, low frustration tolerance, guilt and self-blame.

As you surmised from the preceding paragraph, space does not permit a description of each of these. You can learn more about the causes of motivation by visiting your local library. The causes of lack of motivation are complex and numerous. Most likely there are several causes creating your lack of motivation.

Impact on Job

A lack of motivation can have a negative affect upon you, your co-workers, and your employer. With regards to you, a lack of motivation decreases your productivity on the job. A decrease in job productivity, in turn, can decrease your self-confidence and job satisfaction. Decrease in self-confidence and job satisfaction, in turn, can make it more difficult for you to get-up and go to work. Eventually, you may stop going to work all together and quit. With regards to your co-workers, they may have difficulty understanding your lack of motivation. After several attempts on their part to help you without success, they may conclude that you are "lazy" or "passive-aggressive" or "wallowing in self-pity". If they have to work harder to compensate for your slack, resentment may buildup within them to the point that your relationship with them will be jeopardized. With regards to your employer, he also may experience perplexity and frustration over your lack of motivation. He also may misinterpret your lack of motivation as "laziness", "passive-aggressiveness" or "self-pity". He may believe you are using your disability as a means to avoid your work or reduce your workload. Of course, if he perceives your lack of motivation as severe and chronic, he could terminate your employment. This black picture is not intended to overwhelm you; its sole purpose is to alert you to possible scenarios of the negative impact a lack of motivation can have upon your job, depending, of course, on the intensity and duration of your lack of motivation. Use any apprehension this picture may have elicited in you to resolve to try to help yourself overcome this problem.

Solutions

1. Identify the intensity and duration of your lack of motivation by honestly answering the questions in the *Symptoms* subsection of this topic. Also, talk with a trusted friend, family member, or co-worker and inquire of him about his perceptions of your motivation.

2. Try to help yourself by scheduling one or more simple tasks each day; break complex tasks down into simple tasks and work on those.

3. On a blank sheet of paper make a list of the events and experiences of your life that have been sources of satisfaction, enjoyment, fulfillment, or meaningfulness. Spend some time on this task; don't terminate it prematurely. Aim for more than 10 events of experiences. After you have compiled your list, go back over it and look for patterns or clusters of certain categories: Family, Educational, Vocational, Leisure, Financial, Health, Spiritual, Social, etc. Rank the categories from the one with the most events or experiences to the last with the least. Now do solution #4.

4. Use the categories identified by the exercise in Solution #3 to serve as goal cues for writing goals. Begin with category number one; review the life experiences and events that you identified. This category and the events and experiences should help you think of a current goal you can set in this category that will be meaningful for you. Write this goal at the top of the blank sheet of paper. Now do the same thing for each category using a blank sheet of paper for each goal. Now proceed to Solution #5.

5. For each goal generated during the exercise in Solution #4, develop an action plan. An action plan is a set of 3-5 activities you will perform to attain a goal or solve a problem. On each sheet of paper containing a goal at the top, write your action plan directly under the goal. Write out 3-5 activities you will do to attain the goal. Be as specific as you can. Consult with a friend or spouse for ideas.

6. Keep a time inventory for one week. Using an agenda book, simply record what you did in each time slot. At the end of the week, analyze your use of time. Calculate how much time you are spending in your different activities, i.e., housekeeping, eating, sleeping, working, watching television, talking with spouse, talking with kids, etc. Decide what adjustments you need to make in your use of time. Plan next week accordingly.

7. Ask your co-workers for tips about executing job tasks and managing your time on the job.

8. Identify the negative mind-sets that maintain your lack of motivation. Refute the validity of these mind-sets with logic and evidence from your life.

9. If your lack of motivation is moderate to severe and you are unable to overcome this problem on your own after you have tried, consult with your physician for a referral for professional help.

Action Plan

Overcoming inertia and do-nothingness is a demanding task - one that will require conscientious and diligent effort. An action plan will help you be more conscientious and diligent. Your plan of action will map out activities you can do to increase your motivation. In the space provided below, write out the solutions you marked above. Rank order them by the desirability of their outcome and the probability of success for your problem. Add specific details to make the general solutions more relevant to your situation. Write down how you will implement your solutions.

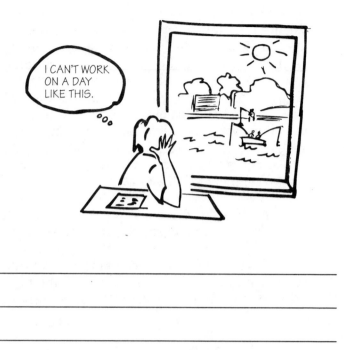

_____

_____

_____

_____

_____

_____

_____

Now that you have completed your action plan, post your plan in a convenient location so that you can refer to it on a daily basis. This will cue your memory and maintain your motivaiton to follow through.

K. SOCIALIZING APPROPRIATELY

Symptoms

Socially inappropriate behaviors are behaviors that do not comply with the unspoken social rules along one or more dimensions: time, age, place, person, content, style, event, or sex. Do you say or do things at the wrong time? Do you say or do things that are inappropriate for your age? Are you overly familiar or seductive with people you don't know? Is your social style of behaving inappropriate for your age, sex, station in life? Do you talk about things that are personal in the wrong places or with strangers? Are your social behaviors incongruent with the social event you are attending (i.e., weddings, job meeting, funerals, graduations, church services, etc.)? Are your social behaviors inappropriate for your sex? Do other people have to frequently tell you what and what not to do? Do others exhibit excessive silence, discomfort, or avoidance when you engage in social transactions with them? If you answer "yes" to two or more questions above, chances are you are exhibiting inappropriate social behaviors.

Causes

There are several possible causes of socially inappropriate behaviors. First, it is possible your memory of social information is impaired. Memory traces for certain social behaviors may have been erased or you have difficulty retrieving the social information in your memory. Second, difficulties with impulse control and disinhibition can cause one to say and do things that are inappropriate. Third, personality changes or severe emotional distress can also negatively affect your social behaviors. Fourth, deficits in processing social information can lead to misperceptions that, in turn, can cause inappropriate social behaviors. Lastly, deficits in executive functioning can interfere with the planning, organizing, initiating, monitoring, and determining of social behaviors.

Impact on Job

Inappropriate social behaviors can affect the relations between a person with a brain injury and his co-workers, employer, and customers. With regards to co-workers, inappropriate social behaviors can be an annoyance, irritant, distraction, or embarrassment. For an employer, inappropriate social behavior becomes a problem when it interferes with employee morale and productivity or if it adversely affects customer business. Usually an employer is unaware of the problem until a complaint is registered. Customers' reactions are similar to those of co-workers with the additional effect of taking their business elsewhere if the inappropriate social behavior is too disconcerting.

Solutions

Below is a list of several things you can do to learn about appropriate social and work behaviors. Read them over. Mark the solutions you believe are most appropriate for your situation and most likely to help solve your problem.

1.   Become a people-watcher! This can be fun, interesting, and informative. Carefully observe the social and work behaviors of your co-workers. Pay attention to their appearance, grooming, facial expressions, and body language. Listen to what they say and how they say it. Use this information to help yourself know what social and work behaviors are appropriate and acceptable. Imitate many of their social and work behaviors. Incorporate these behaviors into your behavioral repertoire.

2.   Ask others around you to give you immediate feedback when you say or do anything inappropriate. Perhaps you can establish a verbal

cue word or nonverbal signal with them that would inform you when your behaviors are inappropriate. Be receptive to their feedback, try not to be defensive, hurt, or hostile. Express sincere appreciation when they give it to you. Apologize for your inappropriate social or work behaviors. And ask the person giving you the feedback what would have been a more appropriate social or work behavior in the situation. Resolve to learn from this feedback and incorporate this lesson into your future behavior.

3. Learn appropriate social and communication skills by reading books and/or attending workshops, seminars, or classes on these topics. In your community there are organizations (i.e., schools, mental health centers and hospitals, colleges, family centers, etc.) that provide workshops, seminars, or classes on all types of social and communication skills.

4. Seek professional help if you are unable to make the necessary adjustments in your social functioning on your own or if there is an underlying emotional or personality factor that is affecting your social and work behaviors. You may need a prescription from your medical doctor in order for your insurance carrier to subsidize these services. Check with your carrier or case manager about the proper procedures.

Action Plan

To decrease socially inappropriate behaviors and increase socially appropriate ones you need a plan. An action plan specifies several things you can do to solve a problem and attain a goal. In the space provided below, write out the solutions you marked above. Rank order the solutions by the desirability of outcome and the probability of success for your problem. Add specific details to make the general solutions more relevant to your problem. Write down how you will implement your solutions.

Now that you have completed your action plan, post your plan in a convenient location so that you can refer to it on a daily basis. This will cue your memory and maintain your motivation to follow through.

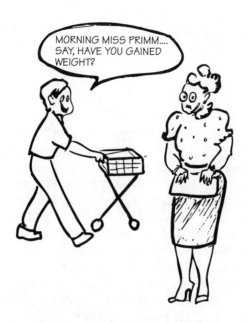

L. SENSING DEPENDENCY

Symptoms

Dependency is relying upon or needing the aid of another for support. During your recovery and rehabilitation process you began to rely upon numerous professionals as well as friends and family members. Gradually you have become more self-sufficient, especially with regards to personal needs and physical functioning. Mentally, however, you may still retain a strong dependency upon others. This dependency need can manifest itself in numerous behaviors. Do you expect your parents or spouse to do things for you that you could easily do for yourself? Do you rely upon others to make your decisions and solve your problems? Do you feel jealous when someone who helps you with your needs is helping someone else? Do you wait to be told what to do and expect others to help you or even do the work for you? Are you smothering a spouse, parent, friend, or co-worker by shadowing them as much as you can? If you have answered "yes" to any one or more of these questions, chances are you are high in dependency need.

Causes

As stated elsewhere in this manual, the trauma to your body also traumatized your ego. For your physical and mental survival you had to rely upon the assistance of others. It was a frightening ordeal. Gradually, you are becoming more independent and less dependent; but, the original trauma may have left lasting marks on your ego. Some of those residual effects are feelings of inadequacy and insecurity. You may not feel as adequate, competent, and secure as before; consequently, you reflexively look to others to alleviate these negative feelings. Another cause of dependency is a lack of trust in one's capabilities. In your everyday functioning you have come to recognize the residual cognitive, social, and emotional deficits you possess. This awareness decreases your self-reliance and increases your reliance upon others for assistance in these different functional areas. Lastly, a pre-morbid (before injury) dependency need is often magnified by a brain injury.

Impact on Job

Here are some ways a need for dependency can affect your performance on the job:

1. You may feel very uncomfortable doing a job alone even though you are very capable.

2. You may frequently request assistance.

3. You may often wait to be told what to do.

4. You may expect others to do your work or help you with it.

5. You may frequently request others to check your work.

6. You may often seek assistance with decisions.

7. You may "shadow" your boss or a co-worker too much.

These are just a few of the many possible manifestations of dependency in the work setting. The major difficulty dependent work behaviors causes is strained relationships. Your dependent work behavior may be time-consuming, physically demanding, and emotionally draining for your employer and co-workers. At first, they might not mind assisting you in any way, but, as your time on the job lengthens, they expect you to become more independent and self-sufficient - maybe not totally - on the job. When you fail to achieve this level of functioning and continue to exhibit numerous dependent work behaviors, they may begin to feel frustrated, exasperated, and irritated with you. When you return to work it is time to become more independent and self-sufficient. This might be anxiety-provoking, but it need not be; you need not become totally independent and self-sufficient right away. You can gradually increase these qualities and decrease your dependent work behaviors by making some effort to do so. The next subsection gives you some ideas on how to do this.

Solutions

Below is a list of several things you can do to help yourself develop greater independency and self-sufficiency and reduce your dependent work behaviors. Read them over. Mark the solutions you believe are the most applicable to your situation and the most likely to solve your problem.

1. Begin by increasing your self-esteem. Go to your local library or bookstore and review books on this subject.

2. Make a point to associate with several co-workers. Do not spend excessive time with just one.

3. Develop external memory aids and cues to help you remember and execute job responsibilities. Rely more upon these external aids than your fellow co-workers.

4. If you are currently receiving frequent assistance, establish a plan to gradually reduce the amount of assistance you are receiving on a day-to-day basis.

5. Recognize your strengths and capabilities. Make a list of them, especially the ones related to your job. Remember that your vocational counselors placed you in your current employment because you have the capabilities to do it.

6. Do not ask someone to do your work. Ask them to show you how to do it. Ask them for tips. Ask them to help you structure your job. Take notes. Write out cue words on cards to help you.

7. Keep in touch with your job coach or vocational counselor. Consult with them for additional ideas for becoming more independent and self-sufficient on the job.

8. If your dependent work behaviors are numerous and/or excessive and you are unable to reduce them on your own, seek professional help in solving this problem.

Action Plan

Cultivation of independency and self-suffiency takes time and action. You cannot speed up time, but you can plan your actions. An action plan specifies several things you can do to solve a problem or attain a goal. In the space provided below, write out the solutions you marked above. Rank order the solutions by the desirability of outcome and probability of success for your problem. Add specific details to make the general solutions more relevant to your problem. Write down how you will implement your solutions.

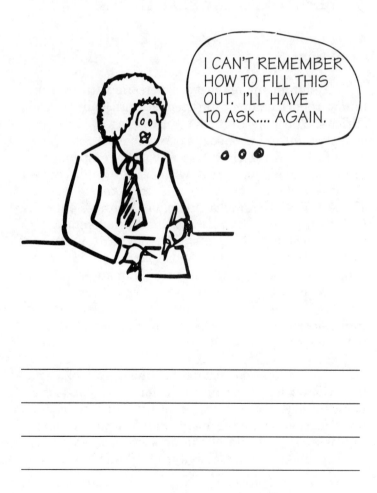

_____

_____

_____

_____

_____

_____

_____

Now that you have completed your action plan, post your plan in a convenient location so that you can refer to it on a daily basis. This will cue your memory and maintain your motivation to follow through.

M. MONITORING MY SEXUAL RESPONSES

Symptoms

A significant majority of persons with a brain injury report changes in their sexual feelings and outlook. You may find that you shy away from encounters with the opposite sex because you think you are less attractive. Maybe you have attempted interactions only to meet with failure and, consequently, you are strongly reluctant to try again. These types of changes in sexual feelings, outlook and behaviors generally are not problematic for the job setting. Nonetheless, they are probably painful to you and your sex partner. This may cause you to avoid all forms of human intimacy, thereby denying both you and your partner a basic need and pleasure. This can increase disharmony in a relationship and lead to other problems if it is not adequately resolved.

The change in sexual feelings, outlook, and behaviors that is problematic for your job is hypersexuality. You may think of little else than sexual functioning and behave inappropriately: making passes at people of the opposite sex, excessive talking about sexual activity, etc. Your sexual interest and desire for engaging in sex has significantly increased. You may be more open and less inhibited in sexually related behaviors. This may lead to off-color remarks to members of the opposite sex, inappropriate touching of members of the opposite sex, excessive sexual jokes and innuendos, and open discussions of sexual matters at inappropriate times or places or with inappropriate people.

Causes

Significant changes in sexual interests, outlooks, and behaviors could be the result of several factors. First, it is possible that injury to the center of the brain that regulates hormonal activity may play a role. Second, injury to the part of the brain that regulates and inhibits behaviors may also be a causal factor. Third, medication side effects can depress sexual interest and performance. Fourth, diminished body image can affect feelings of sexuality. And, fifth, depression can decrease sexual interest and performance. This list describes some of the major causes, but it is not, by any means, exhaustive. There may be other psychological factors involved.

Impact on Job

As stated earlier, decreased sexual interest or behaviors will not generally adversely affect your job performance - at least not directly. Only if you are very distressed over this problem might it indirectly affect your job performance.

On the other hand, increased sexual interests and behaviors have the potential for disrupting your job. The many behaviors described earlier - off-color sexual remarks to co-workers of the opposite sex, inappropriate touching of the opposite sex co-workers, excessive sexual jokes and innuendos, frequent conversations about sexual matters in the work setting are definitely disruptive to the job setting. It is embarrassing for most co-workers to be around someone who is always making sexual innuendos or overtures. The embarrassment, anxiety, discomfort, and insult these behaviors often create can cause the perpetrator to be socially isolated by his co-workers. The obsessional interest in sexual matters begins to be perceived by co-workers as adolescent-type behavior or, possibly, a perverse interest in sex. The most problematic difficulties these behaviors could lead to is charges of sexual harassment. Obviously, a worker who displays these types of inappropriate sexual behaviors is at high risk for termination from employment.

Solutions

Below is a list of several things you can do to help yourself monitor your sexual responses and act more appropriately. Read them over. Mark the solutions you believe are the most applicable to your situation and the most likely to help you solve your problem.

1. Identify if your social behaviors reflect a decreased interest in sex (hyposexuality) or an increased interest in sex (hypersexuality) by asking someone you trust (i.e., spouse, close friend, trusted co-worker) to describe any behaviors you have recently exhibited or failed to display that are related to sexuality.

2. Identify your social behaviors which reflect a decreased interest in sex or an increased interest in sex by observing and recording your own behaviors. Use an index card (3x5") or a wrist counter and place a tally mark on the card or advance the wrist counter one

number each time you exhibit a behavior related to sex.

3. After you have identified one or more inappropriate sexually related behaviors, discuss these behaviors with a trusted confidante. Discuss the possible negative consequences. Inquire about more socially appropriate ways to have acted in place of these behaviors. Discuss current needs these behaviors may reflect. Explore alternative, more appropriate ways to meet these needs.

4. Learn appropriate social and communication skills by reading books and/or attending workshops, seminars, or classes on this topic. Inquire at your local mental health center or community college for information about workshops, seminars, or classes.

5. Modify inappropriate sexually related social behaviors by a) keeping an ongoing record of them on an index card or wrist counter; b) immediately apologizing for them when they occur; c) substituting more socially appropriate behaviors for them.

6. If, through feedback from your spouse or self-observation, you recognize you exhibit a decreased interest in sex, discuss this with your spouse. Inquire about what specific behaviors are lacking. Develop a plan for increasing these specific behaviors in the weeks ahead. Seek professional assistance if together you are unable to resolve this problem to either one's satisfaction.

7. Seek professional assistance if you are unable to modify inappropriate sexually related behaviors on your own. You may need a prescription from your medical doctor in order for your insurance to subsidize these services.

Check with your carrier or case manager about the proper procedures.

Action Plan

Reducing your inappropriate sexual behaviors on the job is a must that requires your immediate attention. You will be more successful at solving this problem if you write an action plan. In the space below, write the solutions you marked above. Rank order the solutions by their desirability of outcome and their probability of success in solving your problem. Add specific details to make the general solutions more relevant to your problem. Write down how you will implement your solutions.

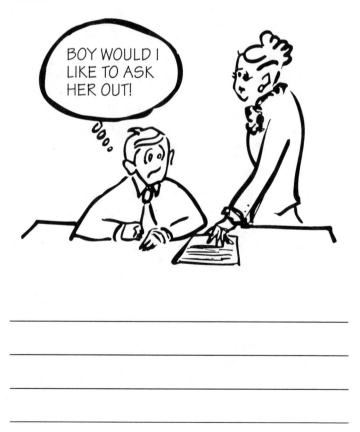

_____

_____

_____

_____

_____

_____

_____

Now that you have completed your action plan, post your plan in a convenient location so that you can refer to it on a daily basis. This will cue your memory and maintain your motivation to follow through.

N. TALKING TOO MUCH

Symptoms

Excessive talking or talking too much means discussing the same topic over and over and over. Do you hear yourself going into excessive detail about a topic? Do you go over the same topic with numerous people? Do you telephone the same person several times a day to the point they begin taking their phone off the hook or turning on their answering machine? Do you hear yourself giving monologues and using most of the conversation when interacting with others? Have you observed others' eyes glaze over or their expression look preoccupied when you are talking to them? Do you often interrupt another when he is talking? Do you feel the urge to say something before you forget it? Do you have difficulty not talking or keeping yourself from talking? If you answered "yes" to two or more of these symptoms, chances are that you talk too much.

Causes

Talking too much indicates a loss of control or an outward display of anxiety. You do this for a number of reasons: a) You may have difficulty remembering that you have already had many previous discussions on the topic; b) you are using numerous talks with others to come to conclusions about your problem; c) you are not able to stop yourself from bringing up the same topic many times.

Impact on Job

This habit of talking too much can be very frustrating for your employer and co-workers. It may make you feel better, but it may not endear you to them. It can quickly become tiresome and boring for them. Pretty soon they may associate these feelings with you and seek to avoid you. Talking too much can interfere with work performance and reduce productivity. We have had employers say that they terminated an individual because he never accomplished anything. All he did was talk all day about what he was going to do!

Solutions

Below is a list of several things you can do to decrease your tendency to talk too much. Read them over. Mark the solutions you believe are the most applicable to your situation and the most likely to help you solve your problem.

1. Identify if this is a problem for you by asking co-workers, friends, and family members if you talk too much.

2. Identify if this is a problem for you by observing your own behaviors and the reactions of

others when you are talking. Do you often hear yourself giving a monologue or sermon? When conversing with others, do you do all the talking? When conversing with others, do their eyes glaze over?, do they yawn often?, do they look away?, do they seem inattentive?, do they try to quickly terminate the conversation and get away? If you answered "yes" to one or more of these questions, chances are that you talk too much.

3. Set a reasonable time limit (1, 2, or 3 minutes) for yourself when it is your turn to talk. Keep your sentences brief and to the point. Remind yourself that in a dialogue you take turns talking. Add questions to your communication to signal yourself to stop talking and signal the other to start.

4. Don't talk to everybody about everything. Decide what topics you want to talk about and with whom each topic should be discussed. The table below illustrates this idea:

Conversation Topic	Audience
Emotional Concerns	Spouse, Therapist, Good Friend
Sexual Concerns	Spouse, Therapist, Good Friend
Financial Concerns	Spouse, Accountant, Lawyer
Health Concerns	Spouse, Medical Doctor

5. Seek professional assistance if you are unable to resolve this problem on your own or if this problem is reflecting an underlying emotional problem (i.e., anxiety, depression) or a personality problem (i.e., insecurity, need for attention). You may need a prescription from your medical doctor in order for your insurance to

subsidize these services. Check with your carrier or case manager about the proper procedures.

Action Plan

Talking too much can be a long standing problem that persists 2-3 years after the injury and - in a few cases - even longer. This should tell you that you have to roll up your sleeves and be serious about working on it. A good place to begin is with a detailed action plan. Use the space below to write out the solutions that you marked in the previous subsection. Rank order the solutions by their desirability of outcome and probability of success for your problem. Add specific details to make the general solutions relevant to your problem. Write down how you will implement your solutions.

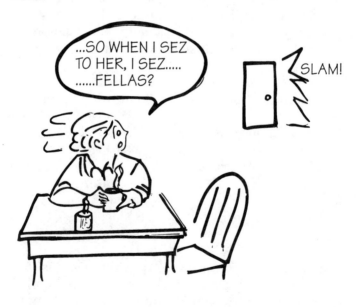

_____

_____

_____

_____

_____

_____

_____

Now that you have completed your action plan, post your plan in a convenient location so that you can refer to it on a daily basis. This will cue your memory and maintain your motivation to follow through.

IV. OPTIONS FOR COMMUNITY RE-INTEGRATION

A. NEUROPSYCHOLOGICAL EVALUATION

During your course of recovery from brain injury a recommendation may be made for a neuropsychological evaluation. Hopefully the person making the referral will explain to you the components of this evaluation. If not, this section of the manual is designed to provide that information.

A neuropsychological evaluation is designed to serve two purposes: 1) to establish a measure of your abilities and skills at this time, and 2) to assist in establishing a rehabilitation program that is ultimately directed toward some form of community re-entry.

What then is a neuropsychological evaluation, and what does it measure?

A neuropsychological evaluation is a series of tests designed to measure brain related behaviors or cognitive functions. The series of tests is designed to measure how well you perform activities that may or may not have been affected by your brain injury. A neuropsychologist may use one battery (such as the Halsted-Reitan or Luria-Nebraska) or a "hypothesis" testing approach (a series of tests grouped according to cognitive skills being investigated) to determine the effects of the brain injury on your everyday functional behavior. The neuropsychological evaluation can well be a long process, so be prepared to spend a day or two with your neuropsychologist.

Specifically, what is measured and what methods do we use to measure the cognitive and behavioral consequences of brain injury?

A neuropsychological evaluation determines your intellectual and academic levels. These are often referred to as IQ and grade level skills. Although IQ scores are generated from the evaluation, the neuropsychologist analyzes the subtest (individual tests within the IQ test) scores as they relate to cognitive/processing difficulties after your brain injury (i.e., you may have memory problems, sequencing problems, perceptual motor speed problems, language problems, or visual perception problems). This information will assist rehabilitation professionals in determining your program and the best situation for returning to work. The achievement test is quite helpful in finding a match between academics and the job situation you may be exploring.

A second important cognitive function measured by the neuropsychological evaluation is memory. The area of memory was discussed in depth in an earlier section of your manual. The purpose is to measure your ability to perform tasks that require some aspect of memory. Three major components are measured: 1) immediate recall - this refers to your ability to remember stimuli, either visually or auditorially, immediately after it is presented; 2) delayed recall - this refers to your ability to recall information (visual or auditory) after a time lag of approximately 20 to 30 minutes; 3) retrieval - this refers to your ability to "call up" information either from a series of repetitions of the same information or from your "long term storage". Your ability to retrieve information is related to your ability to learn new tasks, particularly in the work setting.

A third aspect of the neuropsychological evaluation relates to your perceptual skills. These skills range from your ability to recognize the parts that make a whole (as in a puzzle), to recognizing the whole when you have the parts, to the organization of complex information (reconstructing design without a model). Perceptual difficulties in any of these areas can greatly affect vocational choices available to you.

A fourth aspect of the neuropsychological evaluation relates to your language abilities, including how well you understand and use language, both verbal and written. Your skills in these areas relate to how well you will be able to accomplish tasks requiring following directions, using vocabulary or understanding written or verbal information.

The fifth aspect addresses the neuropsychological evaluation concerning functions controlled by your frontal lobes. The frontal lobe functions are quite important, as they aid us in providing for generalization of cognitive skills to the work place and home. The functions include our ability to continue on a task for a reasonable time or until it is completed, to change mental set (go from one thing to another and then back to the initial, i.e., go from listening to writing back to listening), and to organize complex material and process competing information (reading a book while the T.V. is on).

Lastly, the neuropsychological evaluation addresses the psychosocial or personality changes that may have occurred as a result of your brain injury. You may be asked to answer a number of yes-no questions or answer questions relative to your thoughts and behaviors before the injury and now. Family members can be extremely helpful in providing information about your recovery and changes in family dynamics since your injury.

Neuropsychological evaluations may vary depending upon the neuropsychologist and the questions needed to be answered by the evaluation. However, in most circumstances, they should address the issues just discussed. Many of the activities may be tiring, some may be frustrating, but others may be somewhat enjoyable. So be prepared to sit back, relax, and spend at least one day with a neuropsychologist on your way to your return to the community.

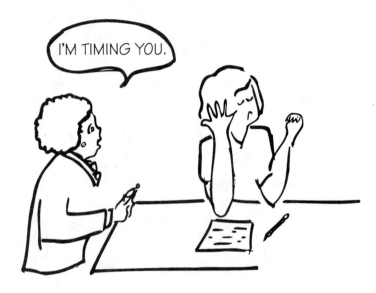

B. COGNITIVE REHABILITATION

A recommendation that the neuropsychologist may make after his/her evaluation may be for cognitive rehabilitation therapy. The goals and objectives for this cognitive rehabilitation program will be directly related to the results of the neuropsychological evaluation. In most cases a separate evaluation that examines cognitive deficits in depth will be used by the cognitive rehabilitation therapist in planning your specific program. As the neuropsychologist attempts to specifically identify the deficits resulting from brain injury, the cognitive rehabilitation therapist attempts to rehabilitate these areas in order to return you to the most functional and enjoyable lifestyle possible. This is best accomplished in two phases.

Phase I of the cognitive rehabilitation program addresses direct retraining in the deficit areas identified by the evaluation. The cognitive rehabilitation program will focus on increasing skills in the areas of attention and concentration, memory, sequencing orientation, problem solving, organization, initiation and follow through. In most circumstances you will work on a one-to-one basis with your therapist in these areas. As you improve you will begin to work on "generalization". That means taking your reacquired skills out of the therapy setting and applying them in either your home or work setting. Here begins phase II of the cognitive rehabilitation therapy.

During Phase II community settings will be evaluated to determine how your cognitive skills level matches with job, home, or social setting. From that point on, cognitive rehabilitation therapy occurs both in the therapy and outside community setting. The primary goal of Phase II is to assist you in community re-entry. The cognitive rehabilitation therapist will systematically phase out of your rehabilitation process and you will be able to maintain your place in the community with minimal support from him/her. Your future role in the community is determined by many factors, some of which are dependent upon physical capabilities, some of which are dependent upon cognitive deficits, and some of which are dependent upon behavioral aspects of your recovery. All of these, in connection with your past work history, and intellectual and achievement level, need to be considered when determining what level of community re-entry (work or non-work related) might be most appropriate.

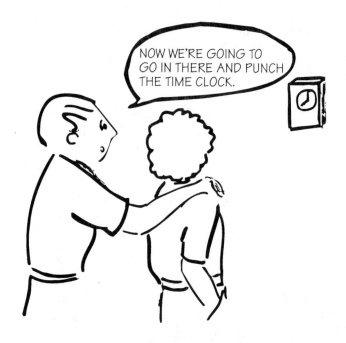

C. VOCATIONAL EVALUATION

In order to better determine the most appropriate work environment, a work or vocational evaluation may be recommended. The purpose of such an evaluation is to determine your physical, mental, personality and motivational capacity, and to correlate those features with existing vocational opportunities. A vocational/work evaluation will also determine which vocational setting would be most appropriate for re-entry: 1) sheltered workshop, 2) structured employment, or 3) competitive employment.

A vocational work evaluation can also determine feasibility for using a job coaching model as you return to an employment situation. There is increasing evidence that a job coaching model is beneficial in every level of re-entry with people who have suffered a brain injury. A job coach goes onto the job site and shadows you on the job until you become independent in handling job responsibilities.

What, then, is included in a vocational/work evaluation that sets it apart from either a neuropsychological or cognitive rehabilitation evaluation? The exact procedure or format used in the evaluation may be dependent upon the individual evaluator or the standard procedure used in a center you attend. There are centers that specialize in vocational evaluation for persons who are brain injured. They would most likely be found in a center specializing in brain injury rehabilitation. That is why information from the neuropsychologist and cognitive rehabilitation therapist, used in conjunction with the work/vocational evaluation, provides us with the most extensive information for your placement.

A vocational/work evaluation may require a significant time commitment on your part. In most cases the evaluation takes from two to five days. During that time the evaluator will look specifically at the following:

1. Physical and psychomotor capacity

2. Intellectual capacity

3. Personal, social, and work hardening

4. Interest, attitudes and knowledge of occupational information

5. Emotional stability

6. Aptitudes

7. Achievement

8. Work skills and work tolerance

9. Work habits

10. Work related capabilities

11. Job seeking skills

12. Potential to benefit from further services

13. Possible job objectives

14. Individual ability to apply evaluation to self

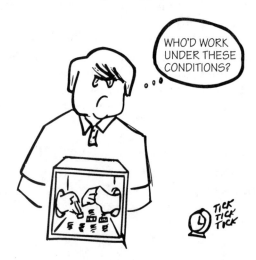

Data are collected in the preceding areas through standardized tests and behavioral observations of your approach to varying situations throughout the evaluation session. The information gathered relative to your capabilities is correlated with the information from a job analysis to determine the best "match" and give you some indication of possible job choices and working environments in the competitive employment market. In many cases, a job coach may still be used to help you use your newly reacquired cognitive skills in the work environment.

As a result of the work/vocational evaluation and neuropsychological evaluation it may be determined that your community (job) re-entry may best be affected through a sheltered workshop setting. In a sheltered workshop setting employees usually are involved in doing piece work for outside vendors. Employees in a sheltered workshop setting are often paid by the amount of work they produce, not an hourly wage. A job coach may accompany you to this setting in order to assist you in completing the job tasks. Tasks in a sheltered workshop setting are repetitive in nature and, after you are able to complete the task, you will be able to work on "speed" and increasing your productivity and dollars earned.

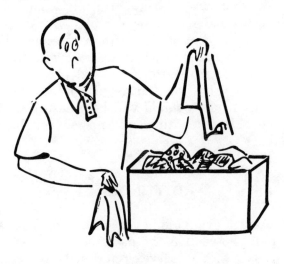

Another recommendation that may result from your series of evaluations is some "structuring" of your job re-entry process. This structuring may include modification in the amount of time you spend on the job during the day, modifications of the particular job responsibilities that you assume, or modifications in the time structures imposed for job tasks. Some larger corporations provide for structured employment within their setting. Positions are developed which have been modified in terms of job expectations and productivity. Again, a job coach may "coach" you while you become proficient in your new work environment. If you were employed in a situation before your accident, your past employer may be agreeable to modifications in terms of hours per week of productivity requirements. This may well be the best scenario for your return to work.

As you return to work, it is best to do so under the supervision of a trained professional (neuropsychologist, cognitive rehabilitation therapist, vocational specialist). They should make initial contact with your prospective employer, continue to follow up with you on the job site for at least six months past the time of your employment, and have periodic contact with you after that. This concept of follow up is extremely important as, unfortunately, many people with brain injury are able to secure a job, but are not always able to keep that job. Consistent contact by the rehabilitation professional will help assure that you will be able to continue in the job you have secured.

D. FUNDING

As you are reading this section of the manual you must be asking who pays for these rehabilitation services. The services outlined are relatively expensive. Rehabilitation costs for people who have had a brain injury can become astronomical.

Funding sources may include private insurance from an existing automobile or major medical policy. Unfortunately, often either the cap is reached or the policy does not provide for vocational or community re-entry services. However, psychological services are covered by most policies and you should be able to avail yourself of the services offered by the neuropsychologist, which would include much of the community re-entry process.

If you were injured in a state with no fault coverage or Catastrophic Care Funds, you may well be able to have your rehabilitation needs financed through the community re-entry process.

Another source of funding can be vocational rehabilitation. They are able to provide for therapies, job re-entry, and evaluative service for clients who are good candidates for return to work. If, at the time you read this manual, you have not contacted your local vocational rehabilitation office, do so now and see what funds may be available to you.

An excellent source of funding for brain injury rehabilitation comes from Workers' Compensation. If you were injured on the job the insurance carried for you through your employer will provide for the needed rehabilitation. Workers' Compensation carriers want to assure that you will return to work, if possible, or that a determination can be made relative to the feasibility of your return to work in the future. Workers' Compensation will provide for necessary evaluations and therapies in order to best decide on lifetime care and/or employment issues. Keeping open lines of communication with these carriers assists them in carrying out this task. You should also contact your local Brain Injury Association office. They will be able to tell you what government funds are available at the state or local level.

Since we all so readily identify with our vocation, it is extremely important for us to be satisfied with our place in the job arena. To that end you may have to pursue the different avenues of funding that may be available to you. Hopefully, in your case, it will be as simplistic as using the funds available through insurance. However, if that is not the case, you (or a family member) may have to become an advocate for your future community or job re-entry needs.

Good luck in that pursuit.

V. Conclusion

Like all life's challenges, the world of work can be fraught with obstacles and problems. The good news for individuals with a brain injury is that these obstacles and problems can be overcome! What is needed is to be sensitive to the problems and then be willing to make the effort to change either our environment, the way we deal with situations or our relationships with our co-workers. For individuals with a brain injury who intend to return to work or are ready for work, this manual can act as a guidepost to help identify and solve many of the problems that can arise. By following the recommendations given in the manual, you will be taking advantage of the combined experience of the authors' years of successfully counseling persons with a brain injury who are dealing with work related issues.

Most of the recommendations, like keeping a daily calendar, using a tape recorder or appropriate goal setting are simple to do yet can reap big rewards. The biggest road block to success is simply failing to use these techniques - so start now to build these into your daily routine. But don't stop there. Keep this manual and periodically review sections as new problems and challenges arise, often when you least expect them. And remember not every situation is the same, so try not to get discouraged if your first attempt does not bring the best results. No employee is immune from problems on the job from time to time. As you earnestly try to improve your performance, your supervisor/boss cannot help but be impressed at how serious you are about starting (or keeping) your new job. In addition he/she will come to view you with a whole new respect and regard you as a true asset to the company.

Lastly, not every job is the "right one". Like a good relationship, it may take a little trial and error to find the right job for you. So hang in there! In the end, the final good news is the enjoyment you will get from a job well done and relationships you will build with new friends and co-workers.

Western
Forbes

1493787

CPSIA information can be obtained
at www.ICGtesting.com
Printed in the USA
LVOW13s1910231117
557352LV00028B/190/P

9 781941 052